THE

Art

OF

Acupuncture Techniques

Robert Johns

The Art of Acupuncture Techniques

Copyright © 1996 by Robert Johns.

Published by
North Atlantic Books
P.O. Box 12327
Berkeley, California 94712

Cover art and paintings of the four seasons by Dr. Andrew E. Tseng.
Book design by Lazarus Productions.
Cover design by Legacy Media, Inc.
Photography by James Lerager.
Special acknowledgment to Mary Harper, Ph.D., founder and director of Changing Systems; and to Elizabeth Kim for their editorial contributions.

The Art of Acupuncture Techniques is sponsored by the Society for the Study of Native Arts and Sciences, a nonprofit educational corporation whose goals are to develop an educational and crosscultural perspective linking various scientific, social, and artistic fields; to nurture a holistic view of the arts, sciences, humanities, and healing; and to publish and distribute literature on the relationship of mind, body, and nature.

Library of Congress Cataloging-in-Publication Data

Johns, Robert, 1945–
 The art of acupuncture techniques / Robert Johns.
  p. cm.
 Includes index.
 ISBN 1-55643-230-5
 1. Acupuncture   I. Title.
 [DNLM: 1. Acupuncture Therapy. 2. Acupuncture Points. WB 369
J65a 1996]
RM184.J64 1996
615.8'92--dc20
DNLM/DLC
for Library of Congress   96-27949
                                                              CIP

DEDICATED

to

Dr. Andrew E. Tseng,

whose teaching and guidance

provided the material for this book.

Romanization of Chinese words in the text is in *Pinyin,*
the system currently used in mainland China.

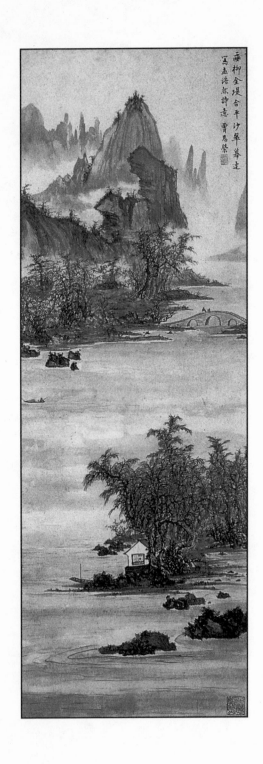

art (ärt) *n.* Human effort to imitate, supplement,

alter, or counteract the work of nature.

American Heritage Dictionary

"Art is a curious, ill-defined, and elusive combination

of craft and invention."

Richard Rhodes
How to Write

viii •

TABLE OF CONTENTS

Preface

The ideas presented in this book come from more than a decade of apprenticeship with Dr. Andrew E. Tseng, a former District Physician of Shanghai during the 1950s and early 1960s. Before his retirement, Dr. Tseng was a clinician at the Haight-Ashbury Free Clinic, and was the senior clinical and didactic instructor at the San Francisco College of Acupuncture and Oriental Medicine. Through such a long apprenticeship, I have been able to accumulate a large body of knowledge and arrange it into a format accessible to the Western mind. In my experience, this type of translation is helpful to a better understanding and application of traditional Chinese acupuncture since it provides a more intricate and comprehensive framework.

One essential feature of classical Chinese medicine is that the context out of which a health condition arises gives meaning to the whole set of symptomatology and treatment. Changes in the emphasis of study in modern times have brought about a loss of the kinds of subtlety and nuance that increase the definition and clarity of understanding, and that in turn support a more fully integrated treatment approach.

Acupuncture is not a cut-and-dried linear modality. It is a nonlinear process influenced by all mutually existing factors. Seeing Chinese medicine in this way, as a medical art, helps the reader gain a sense of its multidimensionality and myriad possibilities. It is worthwhile to have the basic subtleties in mind in order to see what can be done with all the possible approaches. A practitioner standing in front of a patient dealing with any set of symptoms has a number of choices. If one approach does not work well enough, other methods can meet the patient's specific therapeutic needs.

Part of what I attempt to do in this version of the classical methodology is to restore the understanding that those subtleties actually do have relevance and effectiveness in treatment. Without them, treatments tend to be cruder or insufficient, and may frequently address the illness only superficially. The classical approach provides a much more comprehensive overview. It considers the *disease complex* and the general condition of the *patient*, as well as the *complementariness of the treatment* to the patient, while providing more insight about the range of options available and the combinations of those options.

Classical acupuncture is founded on the oldest existing text of traditional Chinese medicine, the *Huang Di Nei Jing (The Yellow Emperor's Classic of Internal Medicine,* also called the *Nei Jing).* There are many different schools of thought and practice, all linked to some degree to the *Nei Jing.* However, not all practitioners follow the *Nei Jing* strictly. Some have departed from it by adding ideas of their own. Others have elected not to do anything different but have omitted guidelines. For example, some modern practitioners place little, if any, emphasis on application of needling techniques.

The classical style of acupuncture is based on the lineage of practitioners who have conformed completely to principles of practice established by the *Nei Jing*. This style and practice of Chinese medicine is linked to its roots in the past, yet is not restricted by them. New insights and developments in treatment are always welcome and encouraged; any progress needs only to conform with the classical style by being in accord with the *Nei Jing*.

One reason that information about varied and subtle dimensions of acupuncture is missing from our learning in the West is changes in scholarship brought about by China's Cultural Revolution (1966-1976). The social upheaval that occurred during the Cultural Revolution closed schools and abridged the Chinese curriculum, suppressing scholarship, even to the point that episodes of book burning occurred. As a result, the scope of training in Chinese medicine was reduced to an abbreviated version that was intended to replace the all-encompassing wholeness of the classical style.

Another reason that significant information is missing from the current Western educational framework is that *structure of the treatment plan* and *formal rules of treatment procedure* have historically been taught to a great degree through guided clinical experience. Treatment plans and rules often are inferred rather than expressed directly, with the synthesis of accumulated curative experiences implicitly providing the procedural framework for treatment.

For Westerners, this open-ended and less structured style of learning can be frustrating because at times it leaves much unsaid and lacks explicit direction. The value of such a supervisory clinical approach is that it does not impose rigid conformity. This kind of procedural framework allows practitioners great freedom to draw upon their own experiences and conclusions in forming a treatment plan.

Finally, not many Western students are fortunate enough to learn Chinese medicine through apprenticeship with a master practitioner. This method of transferring the "secrets" of Chinese acupuncture through the oral tradition lies at the heart of the classical style and is largely missing from the Western educational methodology. Our current curriculum in the West requires clinical study to obtain licensure, yet it lacks the extensive training that comes from the prolonged and personal relationship between mentor and student.

Topics in some sections of this book may be discussed more than once, each time from a different vantage point. Even though a problem or set of symptoms may have already been examined, there are varying contextual influences on any given pattern of treatment. These contextual influences in fact alter the pattern of treatment. In the overview, it is my intent to show the reader how the treatment can evolve depending on *context*.

This book is intended as a guide for acupuncturists and for students of acupuncture who have completed at least basic courses in traditional medical theory and in the location and applications of acupuncture points. Students will find this information more meaningful if they are involved in clinical study, even if only to observe, and also if they themselves regularly receive acupuncture treatment.

Additionally, a growing number of people who are considering acupuncture as a therapy may be interested in the text's practical overview of the medical framework and potential of acupuncture. I believe one of the reasons acupuncture is of increasing interest as an approach to healing is that it encourages patients to participate in their own therapy. Patients can contribute to the progress of their treatment—as well as promote well-being in the absence of disease—with modalities such as self massage or moxibustion.

My own experience is that patients who choose to involve themselves in their treatment also wish to be better informed about what they are experiencing and why. In fact, all of the theoretical material in this book has been utilized and explained at some time during consultations in my clinic to better assist patients' understanding. The more understanding my patients have, the more they become involved in the treatment process.

Regardless of whether the reader is or is not in the field of acupuncture, the author assumes a certain level of knowledge of Chinese medicine. This book will occasionally refer to modes of therapy, such as cupping, or will refer to basic pulses, with little or no explanation. For readers who require more information on these fundamental aspects of treatment and diagnosis, many good basic texts are available in English.

It is with deep gratitude that I have been able to draw on Dr. Tseng's excellent mentoring to provide the next generation of practitioners with the accumulated wisdom of his years of practice and understanding of classical acupuncture.

PART I

OVERVIEW

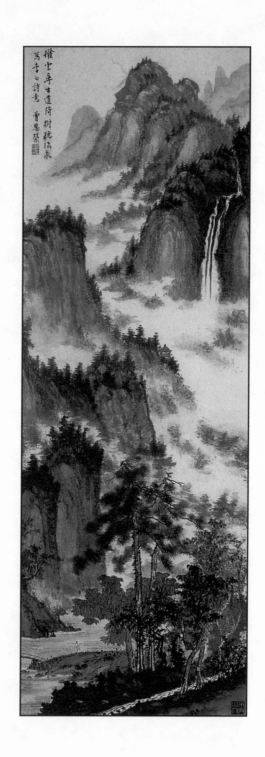

*"You can study medical texts for ten years
and find no such patients in the clinic.
You can work in the clinic for ten years and
find no such patients in any medical book."*

Dr. Andrew E. Tseng

1

A Brief Review of Acupuncture Treatment

There are different facets to acupuncture therapy, acupuncture techniques one among them. These various facets of treatment—diagnosis, point prescription, and methods of administering treatment—are customarily studied separately to facilitate learning them. Nonetheless, it is helpful to keep in mind that in actual practice these facets of therapy do not divide or fragment, but interface with each other as unified parts of a process. For that reason, it is appropriate that a discussion of acupuncture techniques takes into account the context of the other elements of treatment.

Right Diagnosis

In treating diseases with acupuncture and moxibustion, the whole body must be considered. Beyond the patient's chief complaint and the symptoms associated with it, the first consideration in diagnosis is the patient's general strength and whole body condition. With that in mind, treatments for different patients can vary greatly even though the outward symptoms which are being treated are the same.

Since the treatment plan that is selected relies on the findings of the diagnosis, there must be the determination to diagnose and differentiate the *essential* from the *secondary symptoms*, to distinguish the main cause of the disease (the "root") from the signs and symptoms of the disease (the "branch").

Which should be treated first, root or branch? There is no set answer to this. Treatment priorities are established with each individual patient's diagnosis. The ability to identify and distinguish root and branch indicates a *clear diagnosis*. With clear diagnosis, it can be determined which of a patient's needs should be treated first or which can be given greater attention. Consider, for example, the treatment of fever. When there is fever with aching, treating the fever first will relieve the other symptom if the fever is the cause of the aching. When there is fever that is not too high, emphasis is placed on treating the original problem, keeping in mind that fever is just a sign of disease and not the root cause. A child's fever can quickly go higher than that of an adult and can be of considerable concern, while diagnosing and treating an adult's fever can be more deliberate, with emphasis on selecting the proper meridian for treatment. Quick treatment for a child with high fever can be critical, and bleeding the *Jing*-Well Points or bleeding the ear apex can lower fever in a short time. When establishing priorities for treating root and branch, greater attention is directed to the problem that is more serious or critical. If the root problem is not critical, more attention can be directed to the branch.

Chronic and acute conditions can be interrelated as root and branch, or they may be simultaneously occurring unrelated conditions. When chronic and acute conditions occur together, whichever is more critical is addressed first. If the acute condition is not critical, treatment of the original problem takes priority.

This thinking also applies when there is both a surface problem and an internal problem. If a surface condition were critical it would be treated first. When the surface condition is a light one, then some attention can be given to it while greater emphasis is placed on treating the internal problem. As is true with chronic and acute conditions, surface and internal problems can be interrelated as root and branch or they may both be present without having any connection to one another.

This distinctive feature of diagnosis in Chinese medicine, to consider the whole body condition as well as the patient's particular manifestation of disease, requires that many factors be kept in mind. For the sake of practicality, the diagnostic process is usually simplified to the use of the Eight Principles, the theories of the *zang-fu* (internal organs), and the theories of the Channels and Collaterals, in order to locate and diagnose the disease.

Point Matching

Point matching means choosing types of points that match the diagnosis. It is correspondence of the diagnosis with acupuncture points of appropriate therapeutic value. Point matching is general in character. It determines all the possible points that can treat a problem. The points which are actually used for treatment are selected from the larger group of points determined by Point Matching.

In addition to differentiating the pathological condition according to the basic theories of traditional Chinese medicine and then prescribing on that basis, considerations for Point Matching are made in keeping with the peculiarities of acupuncture. For example, treatment of skin problems with Chinese herbal medicine is frequently directed to the Liver, whereas treating the same type of problems with acupuncture is through selection of points on the Large Intestine and Spleen Channels. Another example is the difference between the use of needles and moxibustion. When treating high blood pressure, any of a number of points all over the body can be selected if applying acupuncture. However, when moxibustion is used to treat high blood pressure, just a few points below the knees can be selected since moxa treatment on the head, the neck, the torso, or the upper extremities can cause the blood pressure to rise.

Channel Points

Points are chosen for their therapeutic properties, summarized according to the principle: "The course of a channel is amenable to treatment." This means that points which pertain to the same channel have therapeutic properties in common. One obvious aspect of this is that all the points along a given channel can be used to treat its respective organ. In addition, problems can be treated by channels (interchangeably called "meridians") that run through an affected area. Thorough knowledge of the course of the channels can greatly enhance skills in both diagnosis and treatment.

Matching Points According to Location

Matching the therapeutic properties of acupuncture points with the diagnosis is also based on the location of points. While points on the head, face, and torso are primarily used for treating disorders in their respective areas, points on the extremities treat disorders of both the extremities and the remote areas supplied by their channels. Known as Remote Points, they are considered more powerful and more important than local points.

Problems in the upper body can be treated by choosing points in the lower body and vice versa. Moreover, acupuncture points located below the elbows and knees are very effective for treating the head, the torso, and the internal organs. Points used in this way constitute a style of needling called *Remote Puncturing.*

For problems on the left, points on the right can be chosen or, conversely, points on the left can be used for treating the right side of the body. This is the basis of a needling technique called *Peculiar Puncturing.* This technique is so called because the therapy looks peculiar: while the problem is on one side of the body, the actual treatment is on the other side.

Points Related to Internal Organs

According to the oldest existing text on traditional Chinese medicine, the *Nei Jing, He*-Sea Points and Front-*Mu* Points are indicated for problems with the Yang organs, while *Yuan* (Source) *Points* and Back-*Shu* Points are indicated for treating the Yin organs. In addition, points of the Ren Channel and the Du Channel are indicated for treating diseases of their neighboring organs as well as for treating constitutional symptoms.

Point Selection

In some schools of thought, little or no distinction is made between Point Matching and Point Selection. For those who do distinguish between them, the thinking is that Point Matching means matching types of points whose therapeutic properties correspond to the diagnosis. Point Selection is choosing specific points from the larger number of acupuncture points determined by Point Matching. Point Matching is general; Point Selection is specific. This distinction is made in order to provide more clarity in the final selection of points used for treatment.

Many different elements must be taken into consideration in the treatment of disease. Since *Right Diagnosis* implies a clear understanding, it is through diagnosis that the approach to treatment becomes clear. The standard of practice among some traditional practitioners is that the diagnosis should be so clear that it is possible to formulate two distinctly different prescriptions, each one able to effectively treat the same condition. The ability to prescribe different point combinations for a single problem is made possible by selecting different points from among all of those determined by Right Diagnosis and Point Matching. There are certain benefits to being able to formulate prescriptions in this way. One advantage is that an alternate prescription may be more effective than the one first selected just because an individual patient's response to treatment can vary.

Another benefit of the ability to prescribe in this fashion meets a specific need which provides better quality treatment for the patient. If the patient is being treated daily or every other day, acupuncture points become less and less effective when repeatedly used so frequently; for this reason, alternate points must be found. Traditionally, the ability to draw up distinctly different prescriptions for the same problem indicates a more advanced level of practice.

Point Selection can be explained further through the application of specific types of points.

Yuan-Luo Therapy

Yuan (Source) Points in the extremities are where some of the body's Original *qi* is retained. These points are of great significance in both the diagnosis and the treatment of diseases of their respective channel and *zang-fu* organ. Pressing on the *Yuan* (Source) Points to detect reactions, as well as noting changes in their color and physical appearance, can provide diagnostic information.

For any problem with the internal organs, the *Nei Jing* says the 12 *Yuan* (Source) Points are the most important. The theory is that the Source Points are closely connected with the *sanjiao qi* (vital function of the *sanjiao*). The *sanjiao* is the pathway by which the *yuan qi* (Original *qi*) travels throughout the body. When an area of the body is diseased, *yuan qi* goes into the affected area to promote healing.

Each of the Twelve Regular Channels has a collateral in the extremities called the *luo mai*. Collaterals are the superficial network connecting defined pairs of Yang and Yin channels that are Externally–Internally related. This connection of specific pairs of interrelated Yang and Yin organs, such as the Large Intestine and the Lung for example, is known as *biao-li* ("External-Internal") relationship. "External" relates to Yang and "Internal" to Yin. The *Luo* (Connecting) Points are used to treat diseases which involve two Externally-Internally related channels. They also treat diseases in the areas supplied by two *biao-li* related channels.

Yuan-Luo Therapy involves selecting the *Yuan* (Source) Point on one meridian coupled with the *Luo* (Connecting) Point of its related *biao-li* meridian. Traditionally the method of selecting points has been to choose the *Yuan* Point of the affected meridian or organ, that is, the one which is associated with the root cause of the problem. The *Luo* Point is selected on the meridian that is secondarily affected.

An example of this type of treatment would be selecting the *Yuan* Point of the Kidney, *Taixi* Kidney 3, for low back pain due to weakness of the Kidney, and adding the *Luo* of the Urinary Bladder, *Feiyang* Urinary Bladder 58, for a secondary complication in the legs: weakness, walking problems, pain, or tightness.

Another instance of this type of treatment is one used when treating a problem associated with asthma. Diminished capability of the Lung's dispersing function creates dryness, and it is not uncommon to see constipation as a result. At such times the patient will experience more difficulty in breathing. Since the breathing difficulty is caused by the constipation rather than by the Lung directly, an appropriate and effective prescription in this case is combination of the *Yuan* Point of the Large Intestine, Large Intestine 4 *Hegu,* with the *Luo* Point of the Lung, *Lieque* Lung 7.

Yin-Yang Therapy

It is said that the Back-*Shu* Points along the Urinary Bladder meridian are where the *qi* of the respective *zang-fu* organs is infused. *"Shu"* means "to infuse," "to fill." What this means in actual practice is that the *qi* transports from the Back-*Shu* Point to infuse directly into its respective organ. The back and the upper portion of the body are Yang, and the *Nei Jing* advises that points in Yang areas are appropriate for treating the Yin organs and their respective sensory organs. This treatment principle is known as "Yang to treat Yin," meaning that points with a Yang location effectively treat organs with a Yin physiology.

When we consider the nature of the Yin organs, there is yet another reason why use of the Back-*Shu* Points is particularly appropriate for treating them. The main physiological functions of the *zang*, or Yin organs, are manufacturing and storing essential substances. The energetic direction of these physiological activities of the *zang* organs is inward, or Yin. The infusion of the *qi* from the Back-*Shu* Points into their respective organs is also inward, and harmonious with the Yin (i.e., inward directed) activity of the Yin organs.

The Front-*Mu* Points (also called *Mu* Points), located on the chest and abdomen, are also where the *qi* of the respective *zang-fu* is infused. "*Mu*" also means to "infuse," but in the sense of "gathering." The traditional explanation is that the *qi* infuses out from the organs to gather at their respective *Mu* Points. These points are considered Yin because of their location on the body and are considered especially suitable for treating the *fu*, or Yang organs. The theory that applies to this type of treatment is "Yin to treat Yang."

As the dynamic of the Back-*Shu* Points is especially suitable for treating the Yin organs, so too are the *Mu* Points particularly appropriate for treating the Yang organs. The *fu*, or hollow organs, after receiving and absorbing nutrient substances, then transmit and excrete wastes. The direction of this activity is Yang, meaning outward and away from the organ. Because of the distinctive physiological activity of the Yang organs to empty, treatment to stimulate health of the *fu* promotes their emptying function.

Since the flow of *qi* travels outward from the internal organs to gather at their respective *Mu* Points, the gathering activity of the *Mu* Points promotes and supports the characteristic Yang activity of the *fu* organs.

The distinguishing feature of Front-*Mu* Points to gather *qi* from the internal organs is also utilized to *xie* (Reduce) pathogenic factors (*xie qi,* "Evil *qi*"). When *bu* (Reinforcing) technique is applied to a *Mu* Point, pathogenic *qi* will come out from an internal organ to gather at its respective Front-*Mu*. This happens because *bu* technique will induce *qi* to gather at the *Mu* Point. Once Evil *qi* gathers into the *Mu* Point, *xie* (Reducing) technique can be applied, which eliminates the pathogenic factors that have accumulated at the *Mu* Point.

Internal disease is considered an imbalance of Yin and Yang and weight is given to the importance of restoring homeostasis in terms of Yin and Yang. The balance of Yin and Yang regulates the movement of *qi,* and makes the *jing qi* ("Essential *qi*") stable, thereby resisting and driving out pathogenic factors. When there is disease related to an internal organ, one possible form of treatment is simultaneously needling the Back-*Shu* Points and the Front-*Mu* Points of the same organ. More frequently known as Yin-Yang Therapy, it is also sometimes called *Mu-Shu* Therapy. Originally, Yin-Yang Therapy was used only for cardiac pain, but over time was applied to treating problems with all the other organs as well.

The Five *Shu* Points

"*Shu*" means "to induce" or "to transport." Each channel has five points located below the elbow or knee known as the Five *Shu* Points. Following is the manner in which each of the Five *Shu* Points transports its effects from the acupuncture point to other places in the body:

Jing-Well Points are for mental problems, for a stifling sensation or distention in the chest, and for emergency revival.

Ying-Spring Points are for febrile conditions. *Rangu* Kidney 2 is effective for treating Yin Deficient Heat ("false Heat"), while *Xingjian* Liver 2 treats an Excess condition known as Liver Fire. In addition, *Ying* Points treat superficial disorders along the channel pathway, especially problems relating to the muscles.

Shu-Stream Points are used for joint pain caused by Wind and Damp, and for a heavy or sluggish sensation which also is attributed to Dampness. Like the *Ying* Points, the *Shu* Points are selected for treating problems along the meridian pathway. Sometimes the *Shu*-Stream Points are chosen as a substitute to the *Ying*-Spring Points for muscle problems along the channel because the *Shu* Points are not as painful to treat as the *Ying* Points.

Jing-River Points treat cough, asthma, and throat disorders. The *Jing*-River Points treat fever as well as symptoms of feeling cold.

"He" means "combination" or "combined." At the *He*-Sea Point each meridian combines (i.e., connects directly) with its respective organ. These points regulate the *qi* internally and also drive out pathogenic factors. The *Nei Jing* indicates use of the *He* Points for treating the Yang organs. Inferior *He*-Sea Points are considered in theory to be more powerful than the upper *He*-Sea Points because their location is more Yin (i.e., lower), and thus follows the desired principle of using Yin to treat Yang.

The Five *Shu* Points are also applied according to the Mother-Son Law. Mother-Son Law is an outgrowth of a philosophical theory called the Five Phases *(wu xing)*, which was adapted into medical practice and used to describe the dynamic of mutually nurturing and mutually restraining relationships. Although Five Phases theory has found some place in Chinese medicine, it historically has not been the mainstream of medical theory or clinical practice.

A prevalent application of the Mother-Son Law using the Five *Shu* Points is to *xie* ("Reduce") the Son Point in cases of Excess conditions, or to *bu* ("Reinforce") the Mother Point in cases of Deficiency.

Variations of applications of the Mother-Son Law make use of acupuncture points other than the Five *Shu* Points. One example is applying tonic treatment to the Kidney Back-*Shu* Point for treating asthma. The theory in this case is that Reinforcing the Son, the Kidney, reduces the physiological burden of nurturing by the Mother, thus providing the Lung with more *qi* to restore itself.

Xi (Cleft) Points

"*Xi*" means "cleft" or "crevice." *Xi* Points are where the *qi* of the channel is deeply converged. These points are indicated for treating acute disorders, for pain in the areas supplied by their respective channels, and for pain in their related organs. Experience has shown that the *Xi* Points are especially good for any bleeding associated with their respective channels and organs. Practitioners such as the famous Yang Ji-Zhou have also used *He*-Sea Points for indications that apply to the *Xi* (Cleft) Points.

The Eight Influential Points

Eight important acupuncture points have a close relationship with the physiologic functions of certain tissues or a set of organs. These Eight Influential Points and the tissues they affect, or "influence," are:

Chart 1-1.

THE EIGHT INFLUENTIAL POINTS

Influential Point	Tissue
Liver 13 *Zhangmen*	*zang* organs
Ren 12 *Zhongwan*	*fu* organs
Ren 17 *Shanzhong*	*qi*
Urinary Bladder 17 *Geshu*	blood
Gall Bladder 34 *Yanglingquan*	tendon
Lung 9 *Taiyuan*	vessels and pulse
Urinary Bladder 11 *Dashu*	bone
Gallbladder 39 *Xuanzhong*	marrow

When one of these tissues is diseased, the related Influential Point can be combined into the treatment in order to amplify the desired therapeutic effect.

Or, an Influential Point can itself be the most important acupuncture point in the therapy. Movement, according to traditional Chinese medical theory, is related to tendon. When tendons are affected (i.e., movement is restricted), *Yanglingquan* Gall Bladder 34 is needled with strong *xie* (Reducing) technique while at the same time moving the affected area. The results from using *Yanglingquan* alone can be immediate.

Xuanzhong Gall Bladder 39, the Influential Point for marrow, has many therapeutic uses both by itself and in combination with other points. It is effective for raising the immunity, has a significant effect on fatigue or low energy, treats chronic stiff neck, and is used to dispel the feeling of "cold to the bone." For all of these indications, treatment is with the use of moxibustion on *Xuanzhong*. Moxibustion applied to both *Xuanzhong* Gall Bladder 39 and to *Zusanli* Stomach 36 is an important prophylactic treatment for stroke.

The Eight Confluent Points

<u>The Eight Confluent Points are where the Twelve Regular Channels communicate with the Eight Extra Channels.</u> The Eight Extra Channels differ from the Twelve Regular Channels in that the Extra Channels have no direct connection to an internal organ. With the exception of the Ren and the Du Channels, the Extra Channels have neither *Luo* (Connecting) Points nor acupuncture points of their own, but have to "borrow" points from the Regular Channels which they intersect.

Four of the Eight Confluent Points are on the upper extremities, and four are on the lower extremities. Following is a list of the Eight Confluent Points and their associated meridians:

Chart 1-2.

THE EIGHT CONFLUENT POINTS

Confluent Point	Extra Channel
Pericardium 6 *Neiguan*	Yinwei Channel
Spleen 4 *Gongsun*	Chong Channel
Small Intestine 3 *Houxi*	Du Channel
Urinary Bladder 62 *Shenmai*	Yangqiao Channel
Sanjiao 5 *Waiguan*	Yangwei Channel
Gallbladder 41 Foot-*Linqi*	Dai Channel
Lung 7 *Lieque*	Ren Channel
Kidney 6 *Zhaohai*	Yinqiao Channel

Because Confluent Points are the sites where different channels intersect, they are used singly or in combinations for treatments of specific regions of the body served by the channels. One example is the combination of Foot-*Linqi* Gallbladder 41 and *Shenmai* Urinary Bladder 62 for sagging of the lower eyelid. This prescription is effective because the meridians that are associated with these points go to both the inner and the outer corners of the eyes.

Of all the Eight Confluent Points, the one with perhaps the widest range of indications is *Neiguan* Pericardium 6. The name *Neiguan* comes from two words, "interior" *(nei)* and "entrance" *(guan),* meaning that *Neiguan* serves as an entrance to the interior of the body. For a long time *Neiguan* wasn't considered an important point, so not much emphasis was put on its use. Originally its indications were for treating the Heart, the Stomach, and the chest, but understanding of *Neiguan's* uses have continued to grow, mainly within the last four hundred years. Experience and research have shown that *Neiguan's* connection with many different body functions is so remarkable that it can be used to enhance the therapeutic value of any point prescription. Pericardium 6 also expands the number of different conditions which other acupuncture points can treat, so simple and useful prescriptions with *Neiguan* seem almost endless. Following are just a few examples:

Rapid heartbeat: *Neiguan* plus Heart 7 *Shenmen.*

Atrioventricular fibrillation: *Neiguan* and Heart 5 *Tongli.* "*Tongli*" in Chinese means "unblock the terrain," or "open the land." The cause of fibrillation, according to Chinese medicine, is a blockage of the normal *qi* flow.

Cough: *Neiguan* and Ren 22 *Tiantu;* this prescription is also used for chest pain due to coughing, and for dyspnea.

Morning sickness: *Neiguan* plus Stomach 36 *Zusanli;* this prescription also treats and prevents motion sickness.

Intestinal colic: *Neiguan,* Ren 12 *Zhongwan,* and Stomach 25 *Tianshu.*

Ulcer, gastric or duodenal: *Neiguan,* Ren 12 *Zhongwan,* Stomach 36 *Zusanli,* and Spleen 6 *Sanyinjiao.*

Gas poisoning: *Neiguan,* Gall Bladder 20 *Fengchi,* and Du 26 *Renzhong.*

Also associated with the Eight Confluent Points is a field of acupuncture known as *Ling Gui Ba Fa* which uses only combinations of the Eight Confluent Points. Some advocates of this system use other points as well but apply the Confluent Points first. Because it depends on calculations based on the Chinese lunar calendar, *Ling Gui Ba Fa* is complicated and difficult and has few proponents.

Crossing Points

Crossing Points are where two or more meridians intersect. They are used to treat diseases involving several channels or organs. Because Crossing Points are where the *qi* converges from two or more meridians, they treat a wider range of symptoms and they also have higher therapeutic value. Well-known examples of Crossing Points are *Dazhui* Du 14, *Guanyuan* Ren 4, *Sanyinjiao* Spleen 6, and *Neiguan* Pericardium 6.

Crossing Points on the Ren and Du Channels are generally considered among the most important because these two channels maintain and govern the Yin and Yang of the whole body. Ren means "responsible" and the Ren Channel is responsible for helping to regulate all the body's Yin.

Du means "to govern" and the Du Channel helps to govern all the body's Yang. In ancient times these two channels were not considered separate, but one channel, and indeed they share the same physical location for their place of origin. The ancient view was that to say the Ren and Du were separate would also be to say that Yin and Yang are separate, which they are not. This is supported by the basic theory of the five inter-relationships of Yin and Yang: 1) Opposition, 2) Inter-dependence, 3) Inter consuming-supporting, 4) Inter-transforming, and 5) Infinite Divisibility. If Yin and Yang were separate then one could be considered more important than the other, which also is not true. Good health is defined as the dynamic and harmonious interactions of Yin and Yang, while disease occurs when there is an imbalance between Yin and Yang.

Experience Points

Experience Points are ones which have been found through clinical experience to have unique therapeutic applications or have shown themselves as the best point for treating specific problems. These points have long been used although some of them have no theoretical basis to explain their use. Some examples are Kidney 1 *Yongquan* for coma, bleeding the ear apex for sore throat, Lung 5 *Chize* for knee pain, Heart 5 *Tongli* for high fever with inability to sweat, Large Intestine 7 *Wenliu* for swollen and painful tongue, Stomach 42 *Chongyang* for whole body edema, Stomach 7 *Xiache* for heel pain, and Small Intestine 18 *Quanliao* for frequent urination due to weakness of the Kidney. Though Experience Points are used to some extent by all practitioners, it is considered advisable to primarily select points whose use can be supported by traditional theory.

Ahshi Points

Ahshi Points are reactive sites which can occur in the presence of disease. They may have a positive sensation upon pressing such as pain, soreness, numbness, or distention; they may also have a positive palpable indication such as a mass or nodule. These areas may have indefinite locations not related to Channels or Collaterals, thus following the *Nei Jing* description, "Where there is pain, there is an acupuncture point." Use of palpation for diagnosis is not restricted to the area that is pressed. The neck and scapular area can be examined for problems relating to the upper limbs, or the Du Channel and the lumbosacral area can be palpated for more detailed diagnosis of problems in the lower limbs.

Ahshi Points on the body's surface can reflect an internal condition. Such is the case with palpation of the Back-*Shu*, the *Yuan* (Source), or the *Xi* (Cleft) Points. For example, the Back-*Shu* and the abdomen can both be palpated for detailed diagnosis of gastric pain. When palpating, pressing on different areas should be done evenly for accurate diagnostic comparison. Also, attention should be given bilaterally to help detect any differences or similarities that could help substantiate the diagnosis.

Employing *Ahshi* Points not only as local points but also in accordance with diagnosis and the differentiation of organs and meridians can be useful in determining final point selection. When there is low appetite, belching, and a greasy or yellow tongue coat, a likely diagnosis is Gall Bladder attacking the Stomach. If further diagnosis by palpation reveals gastric distention and pain as well as discomfort under the ribs, it would help confirm the diagnosis. Based on diagnostic information found via the *Ahshi* Points, selecting *Zusanli* Stomach 36 and *Yanglingquan* Gall Bladder 34 would be an appropriate prescription. Another possible point prescription would be *Zusanli* plus *Taichong* Liver 3 due to the fact that treating the Liver will affect the Gall Bladder. These prescriptions follow the *Nei Jing* guidelines of selecting *He*-Sea Points for treating the *fu* organs and the *Yuan* (Source) Points for treating the *zang* organs.

Proper Technique

The Importance of Acupuncture Technique

To say that an acupuncture technique is proper, or is the correct one, means that the appropriate technique is determined by the diagnosis. Needling technique must befit the problems and the patient's general condition according to the diagnostic findings. No point prescription in itself is the ultimate answer to a medical problem. For acupuncture points to provide the desired therapeutic effect, the proper needling technique must be applied to them.

One of the greatest acupuncturists since the beginning of the 17th century, Yang Ji-Zhou is responsible for many of the point prescriptions in use today. Some of Yang Ji-Zhou's contemporaries were not so successful with his use of points simply because their technique was not effective enough; the ability to apply the Proper Technique is essential. Consider the following prescription, which is used for two different sets of indications:

1)   **Indications:** common cold, high fever but inability to sweat.

   Points: Stomach 44 *Neiting* with *xie* technique (Reducing);

   Large Intestine 4 *Hegu, bu* technique (Reinforcing);

   Kidney 7 *Fuliu, xie* technique (Reducing);

   Du 14 *Dazhui,* Even technique.

2) **Indications:** common cold, fever with profuse sweating.

   Points: Stomach 44 *Neiting,* Even technique;

   Large Intestine 4 *Hegu, xie* technique (Reducing);

   Kidney 7 *Fuliu, bu* technique (Reinforcing);

   Du 14 *Dazhui,* Even technique.

Needling Response and Maintenance of *Qi*

Needling response *(de qi)* is typified by increased feeling of tightness or heaviness around the needle. It is described as a fish hooked on a line, jumping up and down, floating and deep. The patient's response to the arrival of *qi* may be light or very slow in coming. When the *qi* comes late or takes a long time to arrive, it indicates that the patient is weak and that overall response to treatment will be slow. The strong patient experiences a quick arrival of *qi*. When the *qi* comes quickly the therapeutic results also are quick. Slow arrival of *qi* or a weak response can also indicate incorrect depth of needling or wrong placement of the needle.

The importance of the arrival of *qi* cannot be overstated: in order to apply the desired technique there must first be arrival of *qi,* or needling response. Moreover, getting the *qi* to arrive and then administering a technique is not enough. The presence of the *qi* around the needle needs to be maintained so there is continuity of therapeutic effect during the treatment. If necessary, this can be done various ways such as flicking the needle, mildly rotating the needle, or lightly lifting and thrusting the needle. Also, when there is maintenance of *qi,* it is possible to repeatedly apply technique during the treatment in order to emphasize the desired therapeutic effect.

Depth of Insertion

One concern in applying Proper Technique is whether to insert the needle shallowly or more deeply. The guiding principle is that the depth of needling needs to match the depth of the condition. Needling that is deep when the condition is superficial causes the pathogenic factor to go deeper inward. Needling that is too shallow when the condition is deep will likely not produce ideal results, since the condition has not been met at the proper level.

Although the diagnosis determines the depth of insertion, the depth of the needling is not decided through the diagnosis alone. Final refinements concerning depth can also come according to the patient's response at the time of needling. For example, a weak patient may not be able to withstand the strength of stimulation that can come from deep needling. If so, it would be necessary to make adjustments to the needling depth according to the strength of treatment that the patient can tolerate. Conversely, some weak patients have a dull reaction to needling. For them, arrival of *qi* is found only at a deep level regardless of the type of condition being treated.

Number of Needles

Great attention is paid to the total number of needles used in a prescription. A general guideline is not to insert more than eight needles at one time. Many techniques involve the use of just one needle while other techniques use multiple needles or use one needle repeatedly at a given site. Since the effect of multiple needling techniques is more profound, even more strict attention is given to the total number of needles used when these kinds of techniques are applied.

When treating facial paralysis, it is possible to combine the use of one needle at Stomach 4 *Dicang* with one needle at Stomach 6 *Jiache*. However, the insertion of a single needle from *Dicang* to *Jiache* is considered more effective. Even with needles at Stomach 4 and Stomach 6 inserted so that the needle tips are touching, the *qi* is broken and is not linked as well as it can be with one needle through the two points. This type of needling, called Through and Through Puncturing *(Tou Ci* or *Tou Zhen)* was developed because the relatively crude needles in ancient times demanded that more effects come from fewer needles. As needles were refined over time, more needles were added to prescriptions to meet more complex problems. Still, the thinking in modern times is that too many needles are a waste of the patient's energy and also indicate the practitioner's lack of confidence in obtaining results.

The application of bleeding technique also lowers the total number of needles that may be used. Drawing blood from a point is used to get rid of pathogenic Heat and to remove obstruction, such as in the case of pain or trauma. In addition to removing pathogenic *qi*, some of the body's normal *qi* is lost when bleeding a point. Usually just a drop or two of blood is removed from the acupuncture point and only until the color of the blood that comes out returns to normal. When there is stagnation, the color of the blood is dark as it first comes out of the point; when there is Heat, the color of the blood may be dark or it may be brighter than normal. Extra precaution is advised when bleeding Deficient patients because it can weaken them further.

Placement of Needles

Insertion of needles is according to the meridian that is affected. The *Nei Jing* advises that when needling it is possible to miss the acupuncture point but to be certain not to miss the channel, since therapeutic effect can still be obtained from needling the meridian. Traditional location of needles for treatment tends to place emphasis on the use of Remote, Giant, and Peculiar puncturing.

Emphasis on acupuncture points with locations different from those of the disease condition is based on the theory that acupuncture points located at or near the site of the problem are generally not considered as therapeutically powerful as distal points. This is part of the basis of the theory for Remote Puncturing, which is selecting points in the lower body to treat problems in the upper body, or selecting points on the left to treat problems on the right, and vice versa. Moreover, when needling Remote Points it is generally considered inadvisable to select points adjacent to each other on the same meridian. The theory is that when needles on the same meridian are placed close together in the remote areas, one needle can block the effect of the other.

Both Giant Puncturing and Peculiar Puncturing select points located on the side of the body opposite the location of the condition. Giant Puncturing uses meridian points. Peculiar puncturing uses *Luo* Points or is along the *luo mai* ("Collateral" or "Connecting Channel") itself. Peculiar Puncturing is applied when the pulses are still normal in spite of the presence of symptoms. Giant Puncturing is so called because this type of needling is on the main meridian, the *jing mai*, in contrast to Peculiar Puncturing which is along the collateral, or *luo mai;* the actual size as well as the overall therapeutic importance of the *jing mai* is considered greater ("Giant") compared to that of the *luo mai*.

Frequency of Treatment and Patient Progress

For serious cases or for internal problems, treating once a week is not enough. In China, treatment is typically daily or once every other day, with a break after ten or twelve treatments. Serious health problems such as stroke, epilepsy, or brain trauma require frequent treatment, though it is advisable to treat extremely weak patients every other day rather than every day. Even though acupuncture treatment in the West is usually not as frequent as in China, treatment at least two or three times a week for serious conditions, problems with the internal organs, or chronic conditions, can still be enough to provide progress.

During a series of treatments there may be a halt to the patient's progress, a condition sometimes described as "getting tired." This is most likely to occur when the patient is treated often, such as daily or every other day. When this happens, the patient needs a break between series of treatments. If treatments are as often as from once every third day to daily, the usual limit is ten treatments, twelve treatments if the patient is a stronger type. The typical length of a break is from one week to ten days, though it can be as long as two weeks if the patient is weak.

Stroke patients exemplify what happens when the treatments are in a series of ten with a week's break between each series. When stroke patients are treated with this frequency, they commonly show their greatest response to therapy during the breaks between treatments. It is during the breaks that patients have the time to integrate the effects of frequent treatment.

Another consideration if the patient is treated daily or every other day is that acupuncture points lose their effectiveness when they are used repeatedly in such short spans of time, acting in a manner similar to a sensory plateau. For this reason alternates must be found, and acupuncture points need to be rotated after every three or four treatments.

The practitioner needs to be aware that a number of treatments may be needed to determine whether the patient can even be helped or not. If three sets of ten to twelve treatments show no results, this is considered an indication that nothing can be done for that patient. For patients with acute conditions, a few treatments should be able to resolve the condition quickly.

A condition as serious as stroke can show remarkable improvement if treatments are frequent and also begin soon enough after the stroke. Clinical experience has shown that stroke patients who start treatment within six months after an attack show a very good rate of recovery, while for those who begin treatment no more than three months after a stroke, the recovery rate is even better. In short, patients with serious cases or chronic conditions, and patients who are weak, require frequent treatment to achieve the most beneficial effects.

Indeed, the ideal approach to any condition that impairs health is to begin treatment as soon as there is a sign of disharmony. Best of all is the use of treatment as preventative medicine and for the promotion of good health and well-being.

2
Factors Which Influence
The Application of Therapy

Once a diagnosis has been established, there are other details to consider which influence the administration of treatment. Although the Eight Principles *(ba gang)* are customarily used as guidelines for differential diagnosis, they can also be used to bridge the diagnosis to principles and action of therapy. Additionally, there needs to be a sound diagnostic basis for determining the appropriate length of a treatment, the depth of needle insertion, the strength of treatment, and the number of needles in a treatment. Finally, application of acupuncture techniques can be greatly affected by the specific points selected for treatment.

THE EIGHT PRINCIPLES

Yin	Yang
Interior (Deep)	Exterior (Shallow)
Xu (Deficiency)	*Shi* (Excess)
Cold	Hot

Yin and Yang

Yin and Yang incorporate all the aspects of the Eight Principles. In this way Yin and Yang are very broad concepts that can be difficult to grasp when thinking linearly. Difficulty in clearly discerning Yin and Yang is also due to their infinite shades of relativity. Something that is Yang in one relationship can be Yin in a different relationship. An illustration of this is the comparison of *ying qi* (Nutrient *qi*) in two different relationships. *Ying qi* circulates within the meridians and the blood vessels. It functions both to produce blood and to circulate with it, providing nourishment to the viscera in the process. Blood is more substantial, while *qi* is more subtle; blood is passive and relies on the activity of *qi* to produce it and to move it. By comparison, *ying qi* is more Yang than blood. On the other hand, *ying qi* is more internal than *wei qi* (Defensive *qi*). *Wei qi* circulates outside the meridians and blood vessels and is mainly distributed in the muscles and skin to warm and nourish the subcutaneous tissues, controls the opening and closing of the pores, and defends the body from external pathogenic factors *(wai xie)*. Internal corresponds to Yin, so the more internal *ying qi* is Yin when compared to *wei qi*. Without any alteration of its nature, *ying qi,* a Yang substance when compared to blood, becomes Yin when compared to *wei qi*.

Because it can sometimes be difficult to view Yin and Yang in simple, direct, and useful terms, a practitioner's ability to diagnose and treat solely in terms of Yin and Yang is considered the hallmark of advanced skill. It helps to keep in mind that Chinese medicine, like biology or physics, is a natural science. By observing and understanding interactions and cycles in nature, we can have a clearer understanding of Yin and Yang. For example, when a patient's symptoms are worse at night, it indicates that the condition is more serious. Night is Yin, cool, dark, quiet, and inward; while day is Yang, warm, bright, active, and outward. Yin is more internal when compared to Yang. The more internal a health problem becomes, the more serious it is.

Consider the interrelation of Yin and Yang in treating chronic cough. A problem with cough relates to *qi*, whether it is *qi* Deficiency or *qi* stagnation, and problems with *qi* correspond to Yang. However, chronic problems are Yin in comparison to acute conditions, which are Yang in character. Acute problems resolve more quickly, while chronic problems respond more slowly.

The Chinese for chronic is literally "slow moving disease." Yin conditions are more difficult to treat because they do not respond to treatment quickly. Also, because Yin by comparison is deeper or more internal than Yang, a Yin condition is considered more serious than a disease which is Yang. So, a patient with chronic cough will require more treatments than will a patient with acute cough. Some patients with chronic cough have symptoms which are worse at night. Since night-time is Yin, coughing which is worse at night is an indication that the condition is even more difficult to treat. It is important that a practitioner understands the rate at which a disease will tend to respond, and does not lose confidence when treating conditions which at first show little or no response to treatment.

Interior and Exterior

Interior and Exterior indicate the location of the disease and also indicate the seriousness of the problem.

The location of health problems may be shallow, affecting skin or muscle, or it may be deep, affecting tendon or bone. Pain which is aggravated by pressing indicates that the problem is deep, while pain which is relieved by pressing indicates the problem is shallow. If pain in the muscle is shallow and needling into the muscle is deep, the result is that the problem goes deeper into the muscle. It is important that the depth of needling matches the depth of the condition.

The depth of a disease also indicates its seriousness according to levels of physiological function. A problem in the meridian is less serious than a problem with an organ, and a problem in the blood is more serious than a problem with the *qi*. Deep problems are more serious and more difficult to treat than problems which are shallow.

Seriousness of problems can sometimes be diagnosed according to their actual location on the body. In the diagnosis of stroke-induced paralysis, it is considered more serious when men have paralysis on the left side of the body rather than the right. By nature, men's radial pulses are stronger on the left side than on the right. In the *Nei Jing* the left is called the Yang side of the body. Men are more Yang, so if the paralysis is on the Yang side of the body, the left side, the condition is more serious than if on the right side. The complete opposite is true for women. Women's radial pulses are stronger on the right side, the Yin side of the body. Since women are more Yin, paralysis on the right side is more serious and more difficult to treat than if it is on the left.

How shallow or deep the condition is determines the depth of needle insertion. For problems on or near the surface, the principle of treatment is shallow needling. If the condition is deep, then the needling also is deeper. Right diagnosis about the level of disease can provide better response because it helps determine the appropriate treatment.

Excess and Deficiency

Excess *(shi)* means that there is an excess of pathogenic factors or that the pathogen is strong. When there is a *shi* condition, the *qi* of the whole body *(zheng qi* or *zhen qi, "*Vital *qi")* is still nearly normal, which is to say that the patient is strong. One sign of Excess is hyperactivity in the pulse. The basis of *xie* (Reducing) technique for treating Excess is stated in the *Li He Zhen Xie Lun* portion of the *Ling Shu:* "When there is Excess in the pulse, go against the condition and take away by force." To take away Excess "by force" means that *xie* technique is accomplished by strong treatment. When taking away an Excess, a small amount of the body's *zhen qi* is also lost. Since the Vital *qi* is nearly normal in cases of Excess, Reducing technique does not drain or weaken the patient.

Xu (Deficiency) means there is a deficiency of the patient's *qi*. This means there is lowered body function or lowered resistance that allows a pathogenic factor to enter. Where there is Deficiency, pathogens may reside, and it is good to keep in mind that even within Excess there is some level of Deficiency that occurs when disease takes root in the body. Typical of Deficiency is weakness in the pulse. The basis of *bu* (Reinforcing) technique for treating Deficiency, according to the *Ling Shu,* is: "When there is Deficiency in the pulse, follow the condition and restore." To "follow the condition" means to acknowledge the patient's weakened state and administer mild treatment in order to restore health.

When formulating a treatment plan based on Excess and Deficiency, the general guideline is: "For Excess use more needles and less moxa; for

Deficiency use fewer needles and more moxa." For Interior problems of the *shi* type, moxibustion generally is not used. The notable exception is an Interior *shi* condition of the Cold type. For Interior conditions of the *xu* type, use of moxa is generally considered better than needling. However, in cases of Yin *xu*, moxibustion is generally contraindicated. The use of moxa when there is Yin *xu* causes complications. First, it can increase the appearance of Heat symptoms. Second, because with Yin *xu* there is weakness of the Kidney, application of moxa can cause the blood pressure to rise. Since the Kidney is the *Root of qi*, it restrains excessive rising of *qi* unless weakness diminishes this function.

Seldom is a case so simple that there is only Excess or only Deficiency. Simultaneous appearance of *xu* and *shi* symptoms may occur independently or may occur as one within the other in an interrelated complex. In such cases, selecting a treatment plan becomes more complex. Nonetheless, in order to *xie* (Reduce) the Excess or to *bu* (Reinforce) the Deficiency, consideration must first be given to the patient's strength and general condition. Applying *bu* and *xie*, and determining the number of needles, strength of the treatment, depth of needling, and use of moxibustion, are all influenced by what the patient can tolerate. In emergency situations, however, it is critical that the patient's immediate needs be met first. It is after a crisis has been overcome that more attention can be given to diagnosing and treating *shi* and *xu* states and the patient's overall condition.

Hot and Cold

Hot conditions call for swift insertion and withdrawal of needles. Hot conditions are Yang, characterized by accelerated circulation, so needles are generally retained no more than seven to twelve minutes. In addition, with Heat there is a tendency for upward and outward movement, so the appropriate needling is shallow. Needle insertion that is too deep or needles retained too long when treating Heat causes the pathogenic factor to be driven inward.

Cold conditions require a longer acupuncture treatment, not under seven minutes and as long as twenty to thirty minutes. With Cold comes lowered metabolic function; therefore a longer time is required for the effects of needling to circulate out from the meridians and into the body. Cold is Yin so it sinks downward and inward. Therefore, needling for Cold is deeper than when treating Hot conditions. Also, when treating Cold, more moxa is used.

Time

Determining how long to insert needles during a treatment is based on the rate at which *qi* and blood course through the meridians. It was discovered through Daoist meditation practices that *qi* and blood move through the meridians at the rate of six *cun* (six Chinese proportional inches) for each complete inhalation and exhalation. Since the total length of the Channels and Collaterals is 1,620 *cun*, it takes 270 breaths for *qi* and blood in the meridians to make one complete cycle of the body (1,620 *cun* ÷ 6 *cun* per breath = 270). The normal rate of breathing is about 18 breaths per minute, so it takes about 15 minutes (270 breaths ÷ 18 breaths per minute = 15 minutes) for *qi* and blood in the meridians to circulate the body one time.

These figures and calculations are the basis for the fifteen minutes generally allotted for duration of needle insertion per treatment. To leave needles in longer than fifteen minutes taxes the patient's *qi* and functions as a *xie* (Reducing) technique. On the other hand, a short insertion time of seven to twelve minutes is lighter because it places less burden on the patient and generally functions as a *bu* (Reinforcing) treatment. With Cold conditions there is hypofunction and circulation is slower, so the time of insertion can be longer—from twenty to thirty minutes. Conversely, since Hot conditions are hyperactive and accelerate circulation, needles are retained for a shorter time. When needles are retained too long when treating Hot conditions, the result is that pathogenic factors are drawn inward rather than expelled.

Depth of Insertion, Strength of Treatment

One concern that must always be addressed when applying acupuncture is the appropriate depth of needling. Chart 2-1 provides guidelines for depth of insertion.

Chart 2-1.

PATIENT'S CONDITION	DEPTH OF NEEDLING
Acute	shallow
Chronic	deep
Superficial (skin, muscles, meridians, *qi*)	shallow
Deep (tendons, bones, internal organs, blood)	deep
Cold	deep
Heat	shallow
Pain	deep
Itching	shallow
Pain aggravated by pressure	deep
Pain relieved by pressure	shallow

When more than one condition is present, there may be contradictions in the depth of needling indicated by chart 2-1. The way to resolve any contradiction is to decide what is most important based on the diagnosis. Also, through experience, practitioners develop preferences as to which approach seems more effective for the given circumstances. For example, patients with chronic problems usually exhibit weakness. Shallow treatment is indicated for treating weakness since deeper needling tends to be stronger and more profound, and weak patients cannot tolerate strong treatment. Chronic conditions are functionally deeper, more "rooted," by having persisted over time, and respond better to deeper needling. Deep needling for a weak patient with a chronic problem is not contrary to the effects of shallow needling if stimulus of the deeper level of needling is not too strong for the patient. Ways to insure that the treatment is not too strong when needling deeply are to use fewer total needles and to use thinner gauge needles for the treatment. *Since different approaches to a specific treatment can be appropriate for different reasons, numerous options are available for any treatment plan.*

Sometimes, deep needling is selected because deeper treatment tends to be stronger and more profound. In chart 2-2, the desired effect from depth of needling is related to the correspondence between insertion depth and strength of the treatment:

Chart 2-2.

PATIENT TYPE	DEPTH OF NEEDLING
Delicate patient (weak, infants, children, elderly, pregnant)	shallow
Strong patient	deep
Excess pulse	deep
Weak pulse	shallow

Additionally, nature plays a role in affecting depth of needle insertion. In harmony with cyclical seasonal changes, the body's *qi* moves to different levels at different times of the year. This is important to keep in mind since treatments are most effective when the depth of needling matches the depth of the patient's *qi*.

During winter, *qi* sinks deepest into the body and patients will typically reflect this with a deeper pulse at this time of year. Therefore, needle insertion is deeper during the winter. In springtime when everything starts growing anew, the *qi* begins its cycle by rising outward—similar to plants sprouting.

The *Nei Jing* describes the bodily *qi* when it begins to emerge during springtime as fine, like hair growing out of the skin. During summer the body's *qi* is most full and expansive, manifested by pulses that are strong and full at the top level of the pulse. So, needle insertion during summer is the most shallow. During early spring and late autumn when the weather is cold, needle insertion is deeper. Moreover, cold and hot weather—regardless of the time of year—will prescribe needling that is deeper or more shallow in correspondence to the weather and the patient's pulse.

During cold weather in the summer, for example, needle insertion would be deeper due to the influence of the Cold.

Chart 2-3.

SEASONAL EFFECTS ON *QI*

Spring — *qi* begins to emerge	*qi* is fine, like **hair**
Summer — *qi* is most superficial	*qi* rises to the level of the **skin**
Autumn — *qi* is not shallow, not deep	*qi* descends deeper into the **flesh**
Winter— *qi* is deepest	*qi* sinks to the level of the **bones**

Chart 2-4.

DEPTH OF INSERTION ACCORDING TO SEASON

Summer	most shallow
Winter	deep
Spring and Fall	not too deep

The location of acupuncture points is another factor which determines depth of insertion. Since Yang is outward and Yin is deep by comparison, Yang and Yin areas of the body are needled shallow and deep respectively. (See chart 2-5.)

Chart 2-5.

NEEDLE DEPTH DETERMINED BY POINT LOCATION

Yang (head, neck, chest and upper back)	shallow
Yin (abdomen, lumbosacral area, hips, extremities)	deep

A few points in the head and neck areas do not strictly follow this guideline. Gall Bladder 20 *Fengchi* is sometimes needled as deeply as one and a half *cun*. Large Intestine 18 Neck-*Futu* is also needled deeply when treating goiter. Ren 22 *Tiantu* is needled up to two *cun*, though the insertion is downward behind the sternum rather than perpendicular or obliquely inward. Insertion at *Qiuhou* (Extra Point) near the lower border of the eye can be up to two *cun*.

Finally, charts 2-6 and 2-7 give brief summaries of different factors and their corresponding influences on needling, such as depth of insertion, number of needles, and strength of treatment:

Chart 2-6.

CONSTITUTIONAL INFLUENCES ON NEEDLING

Body Type	Needle Depth	Time of Insertion	Number of Needles	Needle Gauge
Robust, strong; dull reaction to needling	Deep	Longer	More	Thicker
Small or thin, weak; sensitive reaction to needling	Shallow	Shorter	Fewer	Thinner

Needle insertion that is deep, that is long in duration, and that uses more needles and thicker gauge needles, is also applied for treatment of *shi* conditions and for Cold conditions. Insertion that is shallow, that lasts for a short time, and that uses fewer needles and thinner gauge needles, is also used for treatment of *xu* conditions and for Hot conditions.

Chart 2-7.

PATIENT'S CONDITION   STRENGTH OF NEEDLING

Acute	strong
Chronic	mild
Strong patient	strong
Weak patient	mild
Pain	strong

Generally, treatment for pain requires strong stimulation. Pain indicates there is some blockage or obstruction of *qi*, and strong treatment induces greater flow of *qi*. The *Nei Jing* succinctly describes this therapy as "pain for pain." This means giving painful (i.e., "strong") treatment to resolve painful conditions, keeping in mind that the strength of treatment is relative to what an individual patient can tolerate. No matter what kind of condition is being treated, it is generally advisable that when strong stimulation is applied, fewer total needles are used for a treatment.

Insertion and Withdrawal of Needles

A subtle facet of treatment is the order in which needles are inserted and withdrawn. There is a long-standing practice of insertion and withdrawal of needles in a certain sequence, which is "from Yang to Yin." This means treating the back of the body before the front, and proceeding from top to bottom, defined as first the head, then the torso, the arms, and the legs.

Though acupuncture techniques may need to be administered to points in a sequence that is not from Yang to Yin, needles are still first inserted in the Yang to Yin order. Consider the case of a weak patient who had severe lumbar pain. In order to treat the pain, *xie* technique was applied to Urinary Bladder 40 *Weizhong,* a point famous for treating back pain. After that, *bu* technique was applied to Urinary Bladder 23 *Shenshu* to treat the lumbar region as well as to generally fortify the patient. Pain means there is blockage and, unless a patient is so weak that it is necessary to first fortify the patient, the general practice is to treat pain first. Despite the fact that in this case *xie* technique was applied to *Weizhong* before *bu* technique was applied to *Shenshu,* needles were first inserted into *Shenshu* in the Yang to Yin sequence, then inserted into *Weizhong.* Moreover, arrival of *qi (de qi)* is obtained at each point as needles are inserted in the Yang to Yin sequence rather than later, such as just before a specific technique like *bu* or *xie* is applied at the point.

With very few exceptions, needles are both inserted and withdrawn from Yang to Yin. The most notable exception is emergencies. Points for treating conditions that require urgent attention—such as heart attack, stroke, seizures, bleeding, or fainting—are needled first regardless of the location of acupuncture points that may follow once the crisis is resolved.

A second exception is extreme pain. One example is a young woman who was suffering intolerable menstrual cramps that were intensified due to endometriosis. She was in such pain that she was in tears and could hardly speak. Spleen 6 *Sanyinjiao* was first selected, which brought considerable relief in a short time. After the decrease in pain, further diagnosis determined that the patient could tolerate more needles to amplify the effects of the treatment. Additional needles were then inserted in points on the abdomen and the forearms in succession from Yang to Yin.

Another treatment consideration is *mechanics of insertion* and *withdrawal* of needles. Emphasis is placed on the use of both hands for insertion, manipulation, and withdrawal of needles. The hand that holds the needle is called the needling hand; the hand that assists the needling hand is called the pressing hand.

Any time a needle needs to be inserted, manipulated, or taken out, the pressing hand can be of assistance. Use of the pressing hand facilitates whatever is being done with the needling hand, such as pinching up the skin when needling into bony areas where the soft tissue is thin; or stretching the skin in areas like the abdomen where the skin is loose. The pressing hand is used in vascular areas to press on blood vessels and move them away from the needle, thus preventing the needle from hitting a vein or artery during insertion. Pressing next to the site of needling with the nail of the pressing hand decreases the sensation of needle insertion. Also, inserting the needle against the fingernail of the pressing hand as it presses on the acupuncture point helps guide the needle for correct point location and angle of insertion. That the pressing hand is of great importance in aiding what the needling hand is doing, is evidenced by repeated emphasis on this aspect of treatment by outstanding practitioners throughout China's history.

Withdrawal of needles needs to be done in a way that does not come as a shock to the patient. Before a needle is removed, it should be rotated back and forth lightly to make sure it can move freely. Suddenly withdrawing a needle without first rotating it can have such a strong effect that it may cause the patient to faint.

Point Location and Acupuncture Technique

The specific points that are selected may have some bearing on which technique is used. As points have different anatomical characteristics, applying the desired technique can be restricted by safety precautions or by physical limitations presented by the site of the point.

Points in bony areas, such as Foot-*Linqi* Gall Bladder 41, or points under the scalp, offer very little room for lifting and thrusting of the needle. In the scalp area, for example, some practitioners rely more on various methods of rotating the needle rather than on lifting and thrusting. A few points, like Lung 9 *Taiyuan* and Stomach 42 *Chongyang*, are in bony areas and are located adjacent to arteries.

When needling next to the eye, large turns of the needle are inadvisable in order to minimize the possibility of bruising. While practitioners may occasionally insert needles deeply in the neck area, manipulation of needles in these points is kept to the minimum to prevent inadvertently puncturing an artery.

Needle insertion on the chest and upper back is either obliquely or horizontally downward, never perpendicular. This is done to prevent a needle from touching an internal organ. Deep insertion into acupuncture points produces more profound effects, but for safety reasons it is not possible in the areas of the chest and upper back. The effects that come from deep insertion are achieved in these areas by long horizontal insertion along the channel pathway rather than by deep perpendicular or deep oblique insertion.

In summary, *Proper Technique* is firmly defined by the diagnosis. Additionally, the manner in which a needle is manipulated in order to apply Proper Technique can be influenced by the site of the needling.

3

Treatment Precautions

A discussion of acupuncture treatment is not complete without some important remarks about safety. Although this topic properly comes under acupuncture techniques, it merits being singled out so that it gets the attention it deserves.

In his book *Zhen Jiu Da Cheng*, Yang Ji-Zhou advises that attention should be given to avoid touching bones and tendons when needling Yang meridians, and that attention should be given to avoid touching veins, arteries, and organs when needling Yin meridians. One exception is an ancient technique of needle insertion called *Guan Ci* (Joint Puncturing), which is insertion of needles directly into the tendon where it ends at a joint.

Guan Ci can be applied for tendon problems such as spasm, pain, or numbness, though most often these problems are treated by needling into the affected area without inserting into the tendon. *Guan Ci* is seldom used because it is very painful and because needling into the tendon without damaging it takes skill.

The *Nei Jing* warns that an acupuncture needle touching an organ or bone can cause damage to those tissues. Needling into the Stomach, for example, can create an ulcer. The tip of a needle touching bone can bruise the bone. There is the obvious concern of a pneumothorax if a needle punctures the Lung. The *Nei Jing* underscores this warning when it states that death may occur if a needle touches any of the following organs: the Heart, death within one day; the Gall Bladder, one and a half days; the Liver, five days; the Kidney, six days; the Spleen, ten days; the brain, immediately.

In modern times, we see many surgical procedures which involve cutting into organs and into the brain. *Yet, what makes an acupuncture needle so different that if it touches a bone or an organ it can do great damage or even cause death?*

An acupuncture needle is unique because of the presence of *qi* around the needle (*de qi,* or "needling reaction"). The importance of obtaining *de qi* cannot be overstated, for without it treatment is ineffective. Yet while the presence and power of *qi* gathered around an acupuncture needle can be of therapeutic value, it can also cause injury, possibly even death.

The power and potential danger of an acupuncture needle, as well as precaution against inserting into organs, are summarized in a warning from Dr. Tseng: *"The chest and upper back are as thin as paper and the needle is like a tiger."* When there is *qi* around an acupuncture needle, it has the ability to affect tissues or body function in negative as well as positive ways. An acupuncture needle should be taken no more lightly than a tiger.

A number of years ago in Shanghai an elderly man was treated for Stomach problems. Among the acupuncture points in the prescription was

Ren 13 *Shangwan,* which was inserted perpendicularly. After the needles were inserted the patient was left alone for twenty minutes, but when someone returned to remove the needles the patient was dead. As it turned out, the position of the patient's Heart was very low, which is sometimes true for elderly patients, and the needle at Ren 13 had touched his Heart causing sudden death.

Perhaps another example of an ancient needling technique can further illustrate the power of the acupuncture needle. Many centuries ago, the treatment for severe hiccups that went on for days was inserting a needle perpendicularly into Gall Bladder 24 *Riyue.* After the arrival of *qi,* the needle was then inserted directly into the diaphragm, which could be felt as it went into spasm with each hiccup. The result was that the diaphragm stopped functioning temporarily, thereby causing the hiccups to stop. This technique can be dangerous if the needle insertion and depth are not just right. There is the potential of needling past the diaphragm and inserting into the body cavity and puncturing an internal organ. There is also the possibility of causing damage to the diaphragm.

A few other areas are also considered delicate and are either contraindicated to needling or are needled with great caution. Within the hairline on infants is contraindicated to needling, as are the low back and abdomen on pregnant women. The neck, the region next to the clavicle, and the areas around the eyes are all very delicate. If needling is over the Urinary Bladder, ask the patient to urinate first so as to lessen the chance of puncturing the Bladder. Also, insertion of needles into points over the Bladder is always obliquely downward, never perpendicular. In order to avoid harm or risk, special care should be taken when needling acupuncture points that are close to veins, arteries, and vital organs. In the areas of the chest and the upper back, inserting needles horizontally or obliquely downward prevents the possibility of touching an internal organ.

In the past, before knowledge was available about sterilization of needles, selecting points along the Du Channel over the spine was a special challenge. It was known that insertion over the spine with an "unclean needle" could cause an infection which resulted in permanent paralysis. For that reason the great doctor Hua Tuo developed use of the Hua Tou Jiaji Points as a substitute for points on the Du meridian. Hua Tuo was the first known doctor to needle into some delicate areas that had previously been contraindicated. Yet when it came to inserting needles in the Du Channel over the spine, Hua Tuo was very conservative.

Fortunately, through modern science we can ensure proper sterilization of needles. Because of this, Du Channel points are now used freely while the great therapeutic value of the Hua Tou Jiaji Points is often overlooked in modern practice. The Jiaji Points are excellent for treating chronic problems, for treating internal organs in areas adjacent to the points, and for treating myofascial pain in the neck, back, and extremities. Moreover, the Hua Tou Jiaji have the same therapeutic abilities as their immediate neighboring points on both the Du and the Urinary Bladder meridians, thus making them very effective for treating a wide range of problems.

The *Ling Shu* emphasizes twelve precautions regarding acupuncture:

1)   **Do not use too many needles.**

Refinements of needles over the past 1,800 years have made possible an increase in the number of needles allowed in a treatment. This has led to use of more needles for treating complex conditions or for treating more than one condition simultaneously. Ancient prescriptions consisted of one to four needles. The current view is to insert no more than eight needles at once.

Even though refinements of acupuncture needles have allowed the use of more needles per treatment than in ancient times, this advice from the *Ling Shu* remains valid. Too many needles in a treatment places an unnecessary burden on the patient's *qi* and can actually lower the effectiveness of the treatment.

Also, use of too many needles can indicate a practitioner's lack of confidence in obtaining results. When there is *Right Diagnosis,* good *Point Selection,* and skillful delivery of *Proper Technique,* then fewer needles need be used for treatment.

The precaution regarding number of needles per treatment also applies to the number of needles inserted into the same meridian. This is because one needle has an effect on the whole meridian. Too many needles inserted into the same meridian can lead to needles blocking the effects of one another. This is especially true when inserting needles adjacent to one another in remote areas of meridians, in points located from the elbows and knees to the tips of the extremities. A general guideline is to insert no more than four needles in a single meridian at the same time.

Some ancient prescriptions do apply points next to each other in remote areas of meridians. One such prescription is Pericardium 5 *Jianshi* together with Pericardium 6 *Neiguan* for treatment of tachycardia. To avoid one needle countering the effects of another, the insertion of the two needles is done in such a way that the second needle enhances the effect of the first needle. One possible way to do this is with a classical technique of needle insertion called Added Puncturing *(Bang Ci),* which will be discussed in detail under Multiple Puncturing in Chapter 7.

The Art of Acupuncture Techniques

2)   **Delay treatment for a while after the patient arrives.**

Delay allows the patient some time to settle down. This promotes greater clarity during diagnosis, such as when taking the patient's pulses. Also, it provides the patient with greater comfort when receiving treatment. The more comfortable the patient is during treatment, the more effective the treatment tends to be.

A modern development of the aspect of patient comfort is that Western patients are usually needled while lying down. Patients are most at ease when lying down for treatment, and are less inclined to be nervous. Patients in China are accustomed to being needled while sitting up, a posture which allows for insertion of needles on the back and front of the body at the same time. Westerners tend to be more nervous about acupuncture so it is advisable to have the patient lie down, especially when receiving treatment for the first time.

3)   **Acupuncture should be delayed if a patient has had sexual intercourse within two hours of a treatment.**

Sexual activity a short time before receiving acupuncture treatment can weaken the Kidney energy and drain the Kidney essence. For the same reason, patients should refrain from sexual activity for two hours after acupuncture treatment.

4)   **Treatment for patients who are intoxicated should be delayed.**

Intoxicated patients who receive treatment, or patients who become intoxicated shortly after treatment, can go into shock.

If treatment is considered absolutely necessary for an intoxicated patient, caution is advised and the treatment should be as light as possible.

One example is a patient who had not slept for three days due to the combined intake of cocaine, Benzedrine, and alcohol. He was in such an agitated state that sleep was impossible. He was unable to find any degree of comfort whether he was standing, sitting, lying down, or moving around. Moreover, he had never received acupuncture before and was nervous about it. His desperation to break his negative cycle led him to consent to the insertion of one needle with the understanding that it would be withdrawn immediately if the treatment proved intolerable. The patient was asked to sit, and one needle was then inserted into Ear-*Shenmen* (Extra Point). As soon as the needle was inserted, the patient remarked with surprise that he felt a wave of calm spread over his entire body. The needle was retained for about ten minutes and then withdrawn, whereupon the patient lay down and went to sleep for several hours.

5) **Treatment should be delayed for patients who suffer overfatigue.**
This is also true for patients who give the appearance of being extremely fatigued. Even for patients in general good health, extreme fatigue should be viewed as a kind of weakness and such patients should be made to rest up to half an hour before receiving treatment.

This precaution also applies to patients who come for treatment immediately after heavy exertion. In addition, patients should not undergo hard labor or heavy exertion immediately after treatment. Physical strain shortly before or after acupuncture treatment can weaken the Kidneys.

6) **Delay treatment for patients who are fasting or famished.**
Patients who are fasting or who are uncomfortably hungry should be fed lightly before and after treatment. Patients who have not eaten at all and then receive treatment can experience any of a number of symptoms, ranging from nausea or dizziness to profuse sweating or shock.

7)   **Treatment of patients who have overeaten should be delayed.**

Delay for patients who have overeaten can be up to half an hour after arrival. If a patient does not volunteer information about having overeaten, an excessively full or tight pulse provides an indication.

8)   **Delay treatment for patients who are extremely thirsty.**

Provide hot tea or hot water before and after treatment.

9)   **Caution is advised for patients who exhibit nervousness or extreme fear.**

This caution includes patients who have a fear of needles. Patients who are highly excited can go into shock from treatment.

10)   **Caution is also advised for patients showing any strong emotion.**

Treatment for patients who are angry, very sad, or showing any strong emotion, should be delayed in order to let the patient calm down. This can prevent a patient going into shock from treatment.

11)   **Patients who have traveled great distance by foot should be allowed to rest prior to treatment.**

12)   **Allow patients who have traveled great distance by vehicle to rest before treatment.**

Travel can be tiring at a deep level and the effects are similar to those from overfatigue or physical strain.

The *Ling Shu* lists additional precautions worth mentioning. Delicate patients should be treated with added care. This includes the elderly, pregnant women, menstruating women, infants, patients with Heart conditions, and diabetics. With these patients it is advisable to avoid using points which have a strong needling sensation. When treating weak patients experiencing pain, delay treatment to let them rest awhile upon arrival, and use few needles for treatment.

Use of some important points, like *Neiguan* Pericardium 6 for example, present a possible conflict. *Neiguan* alone is very effective for nausea, vomiting, hiccupping, motion sickness, morning sickness, and digestive problems. *Neiguan* is equally as important for treating Heart conditions. It also is an extremely sensitive point for many patients. A less sensitive alternative would be to insert a needle from *Waiguan* Sanjiao 5 to *Neiguan* (Through and Through Puncturing).

Heart patients can suffer a heart attack as a reaction to needle stimulation that is too strong. Weakness of the Kidneys due to diabetes allows the *qi* to be easily uprooted, and treatment that is too strong can damage the Kidneys. In order to protect the Kidneys, diabetics require more breaks between treatments than other patients. Also, the strength of treatment for diabetics should be mild and the number of needles in a treatment should be few.

In addition, patients should refrain from swimming and from taking a cold shower or cold bath for two to three hours after treatment. Such activity promotes the development of arthritis. Taking a hot shower or bath after treatment is okay.

Emergency cases are more critical, possibly even life-or-death situations. Acupuncture points must be selected quickly and treatment must be immediate regardless of other precautions. In emergency situations, use fewer needles than in regular treatments, give mild treatment, and retain needles for only a short time.

It can be said that the first rule of treatment is to avoid risk to the patient. A practitioner is also required to be forthright and certain when inserting needles in order for treatment to be effective. The importance of attaining a balance in this respect is expressed in some advice from Dr. Tseng: "When needling you have to be brave, and you also have to be wise."

PART II

POINT
SELECTION

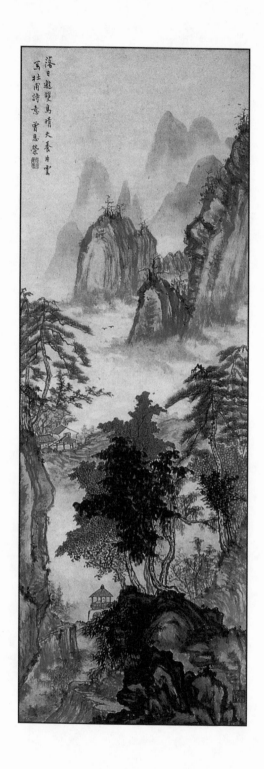

*"Traditional Chinese medicine
is very easy to understand;
it is very difficult to practice."*

Dr. John H.F. Shen

4

Ancient Methods of Selecting Points for Different Problems

Selecting Points by Therapeutic Value

In looking at classical point prescriptions, one of their most remarkable features is the use of few acupuncture points. The first needles used during China's Neolithic times were made of stone and, because these ancient needles were so crude, use of only one or two points at a time was possible. Since only a few points could be used, practitioners had to discover what points were the best ones to select. From a given number of points that could treat a problem, it had to be determined which were the most powerful points and which had the highest therapeutic value. Even in modern times the traditional approach is the fewer needles the better. From the long history of traditional Chinese medicine we have many effective prescriptions which use only two, three, or four points.

Effectiveness of Points Determined by Location

According to the *Nei Jing*, the most important points are from the elbows and knees to the tips of the extremities, on the neck, around the lips, and on or around the tongue. The theory is that these points are more closely connected with the brain, and that these points affect larger areas of the brain than other points. What this leads to is more indications and wider variety of indications for these points.

Large Intestine 4 *Hegu* is a good example. Some of its many uses are for anhidrosis, profuse sweating, constipation, dysentery, headache, toothache, fever, influenza, and amenorrhea. Important types of points from the elbows and knees down are the Five *Shu* Points, the *Yuan* (Source) Points, *Luo* (Connecting) Points, *Xi* (Cleft) Points, and Inferior *He*-Sea Points.

Different Uses of Proximal and Distal Points

For acute problems, the closer the points are to the tip of the extremity the better. Painful points such as the *Jing*-Well Points are indicated for problems such as acute sore throat and *shi* type stroke. For chronic problems, less painful points—those closer to the elbows or knees—are selected.

Hand and Foot Points

Points in the following areas are listed in descending order from the more powerful to the less powerful:

Thumb	Big Toe	More Powerful
Index Finger	Second Toe	
Middle Finger	Third Toe	
Ring Finger	Fourth Toe	
Little Finger	Little Toe	Less Powerful

Points on or close to the thumb and big toe in theory have a wider range of effects. The four other fingers and four other toes are not as powerful together as points on or near the thumb and big toe. Large Intestine 4 *Hegu* regulates *qi*; is used as a calming point; treats low energy, sore throat, and facial paralysis; clears the digestive system; and relieves redness with swelling and pain of the eyes. *Hegu* is a *qi* point in contrast to Liver 3 *Taichong* which is a blood point. *Taichong* is for Liver problems; treats anxiety, insomnia, high blood pressure, and high fever; clears the Lower *jiao*; and clears Damp Heat. Together *Hegu* and *Taichong* are known as the Four Gates, famous for both their curative and their preventative powers. The Four Gates serve as a gateway to the interior of the body. According to the *Ling Shu* the twelve *Yuan* (Source) Points come out from the Four Gates, so the Four Gates therefore help to cover all problems with the internal organs.

Points on the Head and Face

The *Nei Jing* says the 361 Regular Points run up to the head and face and connect with the whole body. A few important points in this area are Stomach 4 *Dicang*, Large Intestine 20 *Yingxiang*, Du 26 *Renzhong*, and Ren 24 *Chengjiang*. Du 26 *Renzhong*, a crossing point of the Du, Large Intestine, and Stomach Channels, is good for problems relating to Yang. It is important as a revival point, and recent research shows that stimulus of *Renzhong* increases oxygenation of the brain. Ren 24 *Chengjiang* connects with the Du, Large Intestine, and Stomach Channels. It balances and regulates Yin and Yang. Du 26 may be used for problems relating to Yang, Ren 24 for problems relating to Yin. These two points may be used together for problems relating to both Yin and Yang, though Ren 24 can be effective enough by itself because it links the Ren and Du Channels. An example of this linking ability of *Chengjiang* is its use for treating chronic stiff neck. Chronic conditions relate to Yin and the neck area relates to Yang.

The tongue is the sensory opening of the Heart, which is the "King" of all the organs. A few important points in this area are *Jinjin, Yuye*, a pair of points under the tongue; and *Juquan* in the center of the dorsum of the tongue. *Jinjin, Yuye* are indicated for speaking problems, digestive and Stomach problems, asthma, and cough; they are very effective for treating Heat or high fever with fluids almost exhausted, such as in sunstroke and apoplexy. *Juquan* is indicated for digestive and Stomach problems, intestinal disorders, loss of taste, rigidity of the tongue, and diabetes. A modern clinical use of *Juquan* has been to restore sense of taste, and sensory and motor abilities of the tongue lost due to nerve damage from dental work.

Du 16 *Fengfu*, Du 15 *Yamen*, Gall Bladder 20 *Fengchi*, and Du 14 *Dazhui* are just a few examples of important points in the neck area. Du 15 *Yamen*, which connects the Du with the Yangwei Channel, is indicated for inability to speak, coma, dizziness, and loss of consciousness. This is a delicate point and needling too deeply here can cause loss of voice or even death. Du 14 *Dazhui*, located at the junction of the neck and the torso, is famous for fever and Heat conditions, treats anxiety, and regulates the Lung. Du 16 *Fengfu* is a delicate point that is closely related to Liver problems such as high blood pressure or loss of speech after stroke. *Fengfu* is also used as a Remote Point for difficulty walking or for motor problems in the lower extremities. All points in the neck have the ability to lower high blood pressure.

Lumbar and Abdominal Points

Some of the important points in the lumbar and abdominal area include Du 4 *Mingmen*, Urinary Bladder 23 *Shenshu*, Ren 12 *Zhongwan*, Stomach 25 *Tianshu*, and Ren 4 *Guanyuan*.

Du 4 *Mingmen* ("Gate of Life") replenishes the *yuan qi*, reinforces the Vital Essence *(jing)*, and strengthens the Yang. It is famous as a tonic point. Moxibustion is used here to increase energy, applied daily for weak patients. For women it is used to treat irregular menstruation and leukorrhea, and this point is well known for treating men's impotence. Since *Mingmen* has a close relationship with the Kidney, it controls the knees and is used to treat weak knee problems. Points on the Du Channel such as *Fengfu, Dazhui,* and *Mingmen* are very effective for treating the extremities. Horizontal insertion of needles bilaterally from Urinary Bladder 23 *Shenshu* to *Mingmen* treats Deficiency of both Kidney Yin and Yang.

Ren 12 *Zhongwan* is a crossing point of the Small Intestine, Sanjiao, and Stomach Channels. It is the Stomach *Mu* Point and the Influential Point for the Yang organs. It is indicated for all *sanjiao* problems and all problems with the Yang organs, strengthens the Spleen by dissipating Dampness, treats flaccid paralysis, and is used for all digestive symptoms. A modern prescription covering a wide range of digestive disorders employs Ren 12, Stomach 25 *Tianshu*, and Ren 6 *Qihai*. An ancient prescription which has been proven to be just as effective uses *Zhongwan* alone.

Stomach 25 *Tianshu* is the Large Intestine *Mu* Point. It is a tonic point used to increase resistance and to treat painful menstruation and irregular menstruation. Stomach 25 is used widely for infants and children since most of their problems originate from the digestive system. When a patient has intolerance to certain foods, *Tianshu* is selected first before other points. Combined with Ren 6 *Qihai* and Ren 9 *Shuifen*, Stomach 25 treats edema or fluid retention. Moxibustion, when applied to Ren 12, Ren 6, Stomach 25, and Stomach 36 *Zusanli*, can stop unchecked diarrhea.

Ren 4 *Guanyuan* is known as the Center or the Root of the body's energy. Because it is a crossing point with the three Yin Channels of the Foot and the Chong Channel, it is an important point for women's as well as for men's sexual difficulties. It serves as an important revival point for flaccid type stroke, revives the Yang, reinforces the *yuan qi*, and restores patients from collapse.

Guanyuan is part of an ancient prescription also known as Yin-Yang Therapy. Moxibustion applied to Du 14 and Ren 4 fortifies the Yin and Yang of the whole body. In modern times, this prescription has been used to treat cancer patients. It has been found that with just the use of moxibustion on these two points, blood values of chemotherapy patients can begin to be restored in one to three days rather than the usual seven to ten days after chemotherapy.

Points On or Near the Extremities

The areas of the chest, upper arm, and upper leg have fewer important points. Points in these areas are better for local problems and do not affect the whole body as much as other points previously mentioned. Important points in the area of the shoulder and hip include Large Intestine 15 *Jianyu*, Small Intestine 12 *Bingfeng*, Small Intestine 11 *Tianzong*, Sanjiao 13 *Naohui*, Large Intestine 14 *Binao*, Gall Bladder 30 *Huantiao*, Gall Bladder 28 *Weidao*, and Spleen 13 *Fushe*.

Of all these points, two are considered more powerful and have a wider range of indications. Large Intestine 15 crosses with the Yangqiao

Channel, regulates the flow of *qi* and blood, clears Yangming Heat, and dissipates pathogenic Wind. In addition to being a major point for the shoulder and upper arm, it treats spasm of the arm and hand. Gall Bladder 30 is good for back pain, sciatica, and for back pain which is referred to the legs. It links the torso with the lower extremities, is used for all kinds of leg problems, and is a very important point for stroke patients with paralysis. In addition, Gall Bladder 30 *Huantiao* helps strengthen the Kidneys.

Other Means of Determining a Point's Effectiveness

Some acupuncture points have a stronger needling reaction than other points and because of this are considered more powerful. This includes all the *Xi* (Cleft) Points. A few other examples of this type of point are Pericardium 6 *Neiguan*, Large Intestine 10 *Shousanli*, Stomach 36 *Zusanli*, and Stomach 37 *Shangjuxu*.

Some points were contraindicated in the past because they are close to vital areas. Because of this proximity to vital areas they are also considered more powerful. Du 24 *Shenting* was listed in an important 3rd-century AD text, the *Zhen Jiu Jia Yi Jing*, as contraindicated for needling. Because the acupuncture needles of earlier times were relatively crude, it was possible to penetrate the coronal suture at Du 24 and cause instant death by touching the brain. *Shenting* is considered the best point for nervous vomiting associated with hysteria. It is a good point for mental disorders and for insomnia caused by fright.

Urinary Bladder 43 *Gaohuangshu* is one of the best tonic points. On the left side it is very close to the Heart and a needle improperly inserted here can kill the patient. The first doctor known to needle this point was

Hua Tuo; prior to the time of Hua Tuo only moxibustion was applied to *Gaohuangshu.*

Experience Points

Experience Points are those which have shown themselves through clinical experience to be especially useful for specific problems but which are not always supported by theory that can explain their use. The following examples of Experience Points are ones whose well-known uses are more closely related to the properties of their respective channels. In addition, these points have been picked as examples because they all share something unique: they prevent disease and strengthen the body by conserving the Root. That means these points have the ability to slow the aging process and thereby help provide greater quality of life and vitality in old age. This can be done through acupuncture or, if the diagnosis permits, it can be done with moxibustion, which is especially good at achieving these effects.

Zusanli Stomach 36 induces the flow of *qi* in the *jing-luo* (the Channels and Collaterals), harmonizes *qi* and blood, and strengthens the Spleen and the Stomach. It is used to treat abdominal pain, lack of appetite, poor digestion, nausea, vomiting, and diarrhea. It is very effective for nighttime incontinence of urine, dry bowel, dysuria, scanty urination, leukorrhea, skin allergies, swelling or lack of strength in the legs, and arthritic pain. Use of moxibustion or needles on *Zusanli* treats shortness of breath. It relieves surface conditions and serves as an important emergency point for heart attack and for stroke. In addition to treating stroke, it can prevent stroke and treat high blood pressure. *Zusanli* is the single most important point for applying moxibustion to strengthen the whole body.

Sanyinjiao Spleen 6 reinforces the function of the Stomach and Spleen, treats all digestive problems, and harmonizes the functional activities of *qi* and blood. It treats a wide range of urogenital problems for both men and women, including irregular menstruation, painful menstruation, amenorrhea, uterine hemorrhage, leukorrhea, impotence, and spermatorrhea; it regulates the menstrual cycle and strengthens the Kidney Yang related to men's sexual functions. *Sanyinjiao* is an excellent point for treating abdominal pain, insomnia, and high blood pressure.

Fengmen Urinary Bladder 12 dispels Wind, dispels Cold, and regulates and promotes circulation of the Lung *qi*. In addition to treating the common cold, influenza, cough, asthma, pharyngitis, and tuberculosis, *Fengmen* is very effective for neck and upper back pain and for treating stroke. Moxibustion on *Fengmen* and *Zusanli* is a prophylactic treatment for attack from exogenous pathogenic factors.

Guanyuan Ren 4 protects the Kidneys, consolidates the Root, and Reinforces the *yuan qi*. It is the most important point for Reinforcing both the *yuan qi* and the Kidneys. Since this point is so closely related to the *yuan qi* it is considered the Center ("the Root") of the body's energy, for all the *qi* in the *sanjiao* comes out from *Guanyuan*. Ren 4 covers a wide range of urogenital problems such as scanty or frequent urination, nighttime incontinence, spermatorrhea, impotence, irregular menstruation, painful menstruation, prolapsed uterus, menorrhagia, delayed menstruation, and itching of the external genitalia. *Guanyuan* treats prolapsed rectum, which often is due to straining during the bowel movement, and also is good for swelling and distention of the abdomen. *Guanyuan* is an excellent point for neurasthenia and for treating high blood pressure.

Quchi Large Intestine 11 relieves surface conditions, dispels Wind, and harmonizes the functions of *qi* and blood. It treats swollen and painful throat, skin allergies including hives, elbow pain, lack of strength in the upper extremities, and hemiplegia. In addition *Quchi* is good for insomnia and high blood pressure, brightens the vision, prevents loosening of the teeth in the elderly, decreases the appetite, and promotes weight loss. It is especially good for prolonged fever and helps treat any kind of menstrual difficulty.

Shenshu Urinary Bladder 23 promotes and replenishes the Kidney Yin. Because of the close relationship of the Kidneys, the marrow, and the brain, *Shenshu* supports the abilities to think, memorize, and concentrate, and in addition helps generate the cerebral fluid. This point treats dysmenorrhea, irregular menstruation, leukorrhea, impotence, spermatorrhea, and either scanty or profuse urination. It treats problems with the spine and low back, and treats diabetes. Since the Kidney is known as the *Root of Life*, Urinary Bladder 23 is one of the most effective points for low energy and general weakness, and it is used for any type of patient who is weak and tired with no strength.

Selecting Points According to Meridians

Selecting points according to channels is done both by specific indications of channels and by indications which channels have in common.

Indications Shared by Channels

The three Yang Channels of the Hand are good for any kind of fever. The three Yin Channels of the Hand are indicated for any problem relating to the chest, such as cough or pain. The three Yin Channels of the Foot treat urination problems, menstrual problems, and difficulties relating to sexual function. The three Yin Channels of the Foot plus the Pericardium and the Heart Channels are for mental problems (whether manic or depressive), for emotional problems, and for epilepsy, which traditionally is classified as a mental problem. The three Yang Channels of Hand and Foot are indicated for problems in the head area.

Areas of the Body Affected by Channels

General areas of the body are covered by more specific indications of channels. The mouth and the teeth are treated by the Yangming Channels of Hand and Foot. Shaoyang Channels are indicated for the hypochondriac region and for the sides of the body. Foot Jueyin treats problems of the genitalia. Hand Taiyang is for shoulder problems. The back and lower back are covered by the Taiyang Channel of the Foot. The Ren Channel is for Deficiency and for collapse, such as *xu* type stroke. The Du Channel is indicated for emergencies such as stroke, fainting, coma, or seizures.

Specific Indications of Channels

Each channel has its specific indications, though obviously the one they all share is that each meridian treats its own organ. The following is a concise list of specific channel indications:

The Three Yin Channels of Hand:

Lung:	Lungs, throat, and chest.
Pericardium:	Heart, Stomach, mental/emotional problems, chest.
Heart:	Heart, mental problems, chest.

The Three Yang Channels of Hand:

Large Intestine:	front of the head, nose, mouth, teeth, eyes, throat, fever.
Sanjiao:	side of the head, ears, eyes, throat, hypochondriac area, fever.
Small Intestine:	back of the head, shoulder, ears, eyes, throat, mental/emotional problems, fever.

The Three Yin Channels of Foot:

Spleen:	all digestive problems, menstrual difficulties, leukorrhea, urinary system.
Kidney:	Kidneys, throat, Lungs, menstrual problems, leukorrhea, urinary system.
Liver:	Liver, genitalia, menstruation, leukorrhea, urinary system.

The Three Yang Channels of Foot:

Stomach:	front of the head, mouth, teeth, throat, fever, mental problems, Stomach, intestinal problems.
Gall Bladder:	side of the head, ears, eyes, hypochondriac region, mental problems, fever.
Urinary Bladder:	back of the head, whole back, eyes, mental problems, fever; Back *Shu* points treat the internal organs.

Commonly Used Points

Points for Diagnosis and Treatment

Acupuncture points which can be used both for the diagnosis and treatment of the internal organs are the Back-*Shu*, the Front-*Mu*, the *He*-Sea, and the *Yuan* (Source) Points. Palpating these points for reactions can provide diagnostic information about the organs to which they are related. Examples of the *Mu* Points are Ren 12 *Zhongwan* for Stomach pain and digestive problems, and Lung 1 *Zhongfu* for asthma and for cough. The Back-*Shu* of the Kidney is good for strengthening the Kidney function and for any pain associated with that organ. An excellent point for both diagnosing and treating the Liver is its *Yuan* (Source) Point, *Taichong* Liver 3.

Interrelated Points

Points are selected from the *biao-li* ("External-Internal") relationship as well as from points related to the affected meridian or organ. Stomach problems due to Spleen *xu* (Deficiency) can be treated by using Spleen 9 *Yinlingquan*. Another example of using Externally-Internally related points is applying the *Xi* (Cleft) Point *Kongzui* Lung 6 for bleeding hemorrhoids. *Kongzui* treats bleeding hemorrhoids for two reasons: first, *Kongzui* is on the Lung Channel, which has a close External-Internal (*biao-li*) relationship with the Large Intestine, where the bleeding is taking place; second, *Xi* (Cleft) Points have been proven to be especially effective for treatment of bleeding conditions.

Acupuncture points which have a special relationship to the affected organ or meridian are also commonly used points. Pain in the area to the side of the navel which is related to the Small Intestine can be effectively treated by using Stomach 39 *Xiajuxu*, the Inferior *He*-Sea Point of the Small Intestine. A similar example that is very effective is the use of *Shangjuxu* Stomach 37 for colitis or for appendicitis.

Mother-Son Relationship

The Five *Shu* Points are selected for treatment both as Remote Points and as points for applying the Mother-Son Law. The guidelines for Mother-Son treatment with which most acupuncturists are familiar are: Reinforce (*bu*) the Mother Point for *xu* conditions, and Reduce (*xie*) the Son Point for *shi* conditions.

There is more to the Mother-Son treatment style than this simple approach; it can involve more than just the use of the "Mother" and "Son" Points derived from the Five Shu Points located below the elbows and knees. One example is *Zhongfu* Lung 1, which intersects with its Mother, the Spleen Channel. *Zhongfu* is considered one of the best points on the Lung Channel for treating asthma.

Selection According to Distribution

Points selected according to their general location are Local, Adjacent, and Remote Points. In general, local points are primarily for local problems. However, any local problem can be in the vicinity of a powerful acupuncture point.

Adjacent Points are those which are relatively close to the affected organ or meridian. *Tianshu* Stomach 25 is often applied for problems with the Stomach or the intestines, and for menstrual difficulties. *Shanzhong*

Ren 17 is one of four Adjacent Points used for lactation deficiency; it also happens to be the most powerful point in the area to treat this problem.

Remote Points are considered the most powerful and have the greatest effect on the head and face as well as on the internal organs. *Baihui* Du 20 is one of the best points for prolapsed rectum and is important for the treatment of any prolapsed organ. This point strengthens the *qi*, treats coma, and is important for all mental disorders, including epilepsy. *Neiguan* Pericardium 6 is famous for treating hiccup, nausea, and motion sickness, and is indispensable for the treatment of any Heart problem. Sanjiao 5 *Waiguan* is a Remote Point for shoulder and upper back problems, and also serves as an Adjacent Point for arthritis of the finger joints and for inability to extend the fingers. Typical point prescriptions are made from combinations of Local, Adjacent, and Remote Points chosen from specific types of points mentioned under Point Matching and Point Selection in Chapter 1.

The following prescriptions are illustrations of Remote Points combined with nearby points for treating different areas of the body and for different organs.

Forehead:

Yintang (Extra Point)

Gall Bladder 14 *Yangbai*

Large Intestine 4 *Hegu*

Stomach 45 *Lidui*

Temple:

Taiyang (Extra Point)

Sanjiao 3 Hand-*Zhongzhu*

Gall Bladder 41 Foot-*Linqi*

Occiput:

Gall Bladder 20 *Fengchi*

Gall Bladder 12 Head-*Wangu*

Small Intestine 3 *Houxi*

Urinary Bladder 60 *Kunlun*

Vertex:

Du 20 *Baihui*

Liver 3 *Taichong*

Eye:

Urinary Bladder 1 *Jingming*

Stomach 1 *Chengqi*

Gall Bladder 20 *Fengchi*

Large Intestine 11 *Quchi*

Sanjiao 3 Hand-*Zhongzhu*

Liver 3 *Taichong*

Nose:

Yintang (Extra Point)

Large Intestine 20 *Yingxiang*

Large Intestine 4 *Hegu*

Teeth, Mouth:

Stomach 4 *Dicang*

Stomach 6 *Jiache*

Stomach 7 *Xiaguan*

Large Intestine 4 *Hegu*

Ear:

Sanjiao 17 *Yifeng*

Small Intestine 19 *Tinggong*

Gall Bladder 2 *Tinghui*

Sanjiao 3 Hand-*Zhongzhu*

Sanjiao 5 *Waiguan*

Large Intestine 4 *Hegu*

Throat:

Small Intestine 17 *Tianrong*

Large Intestine 4 *Hegu*

Lung 6 *Kongzui*

Kidney 6 *Zhaohai*

Arm:

Large Intestine 15 *Jianyu*

Large Intestine 11 *Quchi*

Large Intestine 4 *Hegu*

Hua Tuo Jiaji Points—from Du 14 *Dazhui* to *Zhiyang* Du 9

Leg:

Gall Bladder 30 *Huantiao*

Gall Bladder 31 *Fengshi*

Urinary Bladder 40 *Weizhong*

Gall Bladder 34 *Yanglingquan*

Gall Bladder 39 *Xuanzhong*

Hua Tuo Jiaji Points—from Du 4 *Mingmen* to Du 2 *Yaoyangguan*

Genitalia:

Ren 4 *Guanyuan*

Ren 3 *Zhongji*

Abdomen-*Zigong* (Extra Point)

Pericardium 6 *Neiguan*

Spleen 6 *Sanyinjiao*

Rectum:

Urinary Bladder 54 *Zhibian*

Du 1 *Changqiang*

Urinary Bladder 57 *Chengshan*

Urinary Bladder 60 *Kunlun*

Lung:

Urinary Bladder 13 *Feishu*

Ren 22 *Tiantu*

Ren 17 *Shanzhong*

Lung 5 *Chize*

Lung 7 *Lieque*

Heart:

Urinary Bladder 14 *Jueyinshu*

Urinary Bladder 15 *Xinshu*

Ren 17 *Shanzhong*

Pericardium 4 *Ximen*

Pericardium 5 *Jianshi*

Pericardium 6 *Neiguan*

Heart 7 *Shenmen*

Stomach:

Urinary Bladder 21 *Weishu*

Ren 12 *Zhongwan*

Pericardium 6 *Neiguan*

Stomach 36 *Zusanli*

Liver:

Urinary Bladder 18 *Ganshu*

Liver 3 *Taichong*

Intestines:

Urinary Bladder 25 *Dachangshu*

Urinary Bladder 27 *Xiaochangshu*

Stomach 25 *Tianshu*

Ren 4 *Guanyuan*

Stomach 36 *Zusanli*

Stomach 37 *Shangjuxu*

Stomach 39 *Xiajuxu*

Kidneys:

Urinary Bladder 23 *Shenshu*

Urinary Bladder 52 *Zhishi*

Kidney 3 *Taixi*

Urinary Bladder:

Urinary Bladder 32 *Ciliao*

Ren 3 *Zhongji*

Pericardium 6 *Neiguan*

It is not intended that all the points in the larger prescriptions be used at the same time, but that points appropriate to the diagnosis are selected. The use of only one or two Remote Points is recommended with any of the above prescriptions.

5

Pericardium 6 Neiguan: The Wild Card

For as long as anyone knows, practitioners have added a special point to acupuncture prescriptions in order to enhance the overall therapeutic effect of treatments. In ancient times it was usually a point selected from the Gall Bladder meridian, because it is via the Gall Bladder meridian that the Clean Yang *qi (qing yang qi)* of the internal organs is brought to the head. The Clean Yang *qi* serves various functions, and what these functions share is their location in Yang regions of the body—upward and outward. The *qing yang qi* gives strength to the four limbs, helps form the *wei qi* (Defensive *qi*), and heightens the physiological activities of the five sensory orifices: eyes, ears, nose, lips, and tongue.

Due to this special connection between the Gall Bladder meridian, the *qing yang qi*, and all of the other organs, obstruction in *any* of the Twelve Regular meridians is reflected in the Gall Bladder Channel. Conversely, if the flow of the Gall Bladder meridian is open, then the flow of *qi* and blood in the other meridians will also be normal.

In the early and mid-20th century, a famous practitioner in Shanghai was getting dramatic results treating problems affecting the internal organs as well as any problems affecting the sides of the body. No one could figure out why he was so successful. People who observed his clinical work could not see anything special or unusual about his treatments; he did not seem to use any unusual acupuncture points or any special needling techniques. It was not until after his death that access to his clinical notes provided the answer to his secret. He added *Qiuxu* Gall Bladder 40 to point prescriptions in order to increase the therapeutic value of his treatments. To amplify the effects of *Qiuxu*, the needle was inserted to the other side of the foot, in the area of *Rangu* Kidney 2 (Through and Through Puncturing).

Another point found to function as a central influencing factor in treating many different conditions is Pericardium 6 *Neiguan*. Extensive research by Yang Ji-Zhou at the end of the 16th century on the historical uses of acupuncture points revealed that, in addition to enhancing the effect of treatments, *Neiguan* has a synergistic influence on acupuncture points. In this way, *Neiguan* is like a wild card or the Joker in a deck of cards.

When applying a prescription for treatment, it is possible to bolster the outcome of that treatment by adding *Neiguan*. So, if the results of treatment are not all that are hoped for, adding *Neiguan* to point prescriptions can be a sort of insurance policy for enhancing the healing process in all its particular domains. In a few cases, using *Neiguan* alone may give sufficient results.

Uses of Pericardium 6 alone include treating contracture and pain of the elbow and arm, treating pain or motor problems with the fingers, and treating any kind of fever. *Neiguan* alone also treats cardiac pain, a very serious symptom, and it is one of the most effective acupuncture points for treating palpitation. Beyond the many other conditions that *Neiguan* can treat, its number one function is serving as "protector of the Heart." When forming prescriptions for treating any condition associated with the Heart, it is wise to consider using Pericardium 6. So close is the relationship of the Pericardium with the Heart that in ancient times they were not even considered separate.

Mental disorders are also associated with the Heart since, according to basic medical theory, the Heart has a very close relationship with the brain. A mental problem indicates that something is wrong with the Heart.

Mental disorder in Chinese medicine means that the patient suffers from an inappropriate mental state. This can range from comparatively light conditions like insomnia or nervousness brought on by stress, to more serious problems such as mania, depression, or epilepsy. Diagnosis of the Heart is employed to help evaluate the condition of the brain, and important points related to the Heart, such as *Neiguan*, are used for treatment of mental problems and even for brain trauma.

Neiguan is the Confluent Point to the Yinwei Channel. "Yinwei" means "maintenance of Yin," and main uses of this channel are for treatment of cardiac pain and Heart problems. Blood is a Yin substance, and through clinical experience the meaning of "maintenance of Yin" has been extended to include regulation of menstruation. Consequently, Pericardium 6 is a significant point to consider when forming point prescriptions for menstrual disorders.

Neiguan is the *Luo* (Connecting) Point to the Sanjiao Channel, and facilitates the movement of *qi* generally associated with the functions of each of the three portions of the body cavity *(sanjiao)*: 1) Upper *jiao,* Heart and Lung function to transfer *qi* and blood to the whole body; 2) Middle *jiao,* digestion; 3) Lower *jiao,* water metabolism, storage and excretion of urine, and intestinal function.

According to the *Nei Jing,* "Where there is Deficiency (i.e., deficiency of *qi*) is where pathogens may reside." This means if any place in the body has a less than normal amount of *qi,* regardless of the various causes which can induce diminished presence of *qi,* then that place is vulnerable to disease. The ability of *Neiguan* to promote the circulation of *qi* and provide an ample amount of *qi* throughout the whole body *(sanjiao)* makes it an important point for treating disease and for promoting good health. Moreover, because of *Neiguan's* close relationship with the Heart, the brain, and mentality, *Neiguan* reduces stress and anxiety. For that reason, adding *Neiguan* to most treatment plans will help the patient recuperate faster.

Fifty-Eight Prescriptions Using *Neiguan*

The following *Nei Guan* prescriptions are taken from Dr. Tseng's clinical notes. In using each of these prescriptions, adhering to certain guidelines is advised. Needling points bilaterally is indicated when the condition is severe. When the problem is acute, then strong treatment is recommended. Patients whose condition is chronic generally are not as strong as patients with acute conditions. The weaker the patient's condition, the milder the treatment should be.

1.   **Tachycardia:** *Neiguan* alone. The pulse should slow down within 20 to 30 minutes after the treatment begins. Pericardium 5 *Jianshi* may be added to increase the effect. All points are needled with Even technique.

2.   **Irregular heartbeat**, meaning that sometimes the Heart rate is fast, sometimes slow: *Neiguan* with Ren 17 *Shanzhong*. Heart 7 *Shenmen* can be added to amplify the effects of this prescription.

3.   **Missing heartbeat:** *Neiguan* and Urinary Bladder 15 *Xinshu*. This formula is also applied for palpitation, restlessness, and anxiety, and for the combined symptoms of rapid heartbeat and mild heart pain.

4.   **Angina:** *Neiguan* plus the *Xi* (Cleft) Point of the Heart, *Yinxi* Heart 6.

5.   **Angina:** the needle at *Neiguan* is inserted to the other side of the arm—this technique is called Through and Through Puncturing *(Tou Ci)*— and the tip of the needle touches the other side beneath the skin in the area of Sanjiao 5 *Waiguan*. If the pain is severe, Spleen 4 *Gongsun* is added.

6.   **Heart pain** accompanied by a pale face, indicating blood deficiency: *Neiguan*, Urinary Bladder 15 *Xinshu*, Urinary Bladder 17 *Geshu*, and Stomach 36 *Zusanli* together will fortify the Spleen function to produce blood.

7.   **Chronic heart disease** with a heartbeat that is weak and slow: *Neiguan*, Pericardium 4 *Ximen*, and Urinary Bladder 15 *Xinshu*. The chronic type needs frequent treatment, daily if possible. The stimulus of the treatment needs to be very light.

8.   **Rheumatic heart disease:** *Neiguan*, Urinary Bladder 15 *Xinshu*, and Heart 7 *Shenmen*.

9.   **Hypertension:** *Neiguan* plus Stomach 9 *Renying* can lower the blood pressure in a short time. Great care must be taken to avoid the artery when needling Stomach 9.

10.   **Hypertension:** *Neiguan* and Liver 3 *Taichong*.

11. **Low blood pressure:** *Neiguan* and Liver 3 *Taichong*. Low blood pressure indicates the patient is weak.

12. **Low blood pressure** with sudden tiredness: *Neiguan*, Du 25 *Suliao*, and Liver 3 *Taichong*.

13. **Cerebral Concussion:** *Neiguan* plus Heart 7 *Shenmen* and Gall Bladder 20 *Fengchi*.

14. **Schizophrenia:** *Neiguan*, plus Du 15 *Yamen* and Gall Bladder 20 *Fengchi*.

15. **Hysteria**—phlegm transforms into Heat, disturbing the mind: *Neiguan* and Liver 2 *Xingjian*.

16. **Hysteria** followed by unconsciousness: *Neiguan*, plus Large Intestine 4 *Hegu*, Spleen 6 *Sanyinjiao*, and Liver 2 *Xingjian*. *Hegu* is the master point for the head. It connects with the Stomach and Du Channels, and clears the mind.

17. **Mental disorder,** whether manic or depressive: *Neiguan*, Du 14 *Dazhui*, Du 15 *Yamen*, and Du 26 *Renzhong*. Treatment for the manic type is much stronger than that for the depressive type.

18. **Epilepsy:** *Neiguan* and Du 15 *Yamen*. Gall Bladder 20 *Fengchi* and Du 14 *Dazhui* can be added.

19. **Epilepsy or hysteria** due to Heat resulting from stagnant phlegm. *Neiguan* plus Liver 2 *Xingjian*.

20. **Vertigo, dizziness:** *Neiguan*, Gall Bladder 20 *Fengchi*, Du 20 *Baihui*, and Liver 3 *Taichong*.

21. **Insomnia:** *Neiguan* plus Stomach 36 *Zusanli*, and Spleen 6 *Sanyinjiao*.

22. **Insomnia:** *Neiguan* and Kidney 3 *Taixi*. Kidney 3 is a very good point for the Heart. Points that can be added to amplify effects of the treatment include *Yintang* (Extra Point), Ear-*Shenmen*, and Heart 7 *Shenmen*.

23. Neurasthenia: *Neiguan* with Kidney 7 *Fuliu*. *Fuliu* itself is a good point for a weak Heart; it can make the pulse stronger. The meaning of *"Fuliu"* in Chinese is "return of the flow."

24. Bronchial wheezing: *Neiguan*, Stomach 40 *Fenglong*, and Liver 2 *Xingjian*.

25. Cough with copious sputum, and the patient is weak: *Neiguan*, Ren 22 *Tiantu*, and *Zusanli* Stomach 36. *Zusanli* is very good both for cleaning up the sputum and for making the patient stronger.

26. Cough, asthma: *Neiguan* plus Urinary Bladder 13 *Feishu*.

27. Asthma: *Neiguan* and *Dingchuan* (Extra Point). These two points added to any prescription for asthma greatly enhance the effects of the treatment.

28. Whooping cough: *Neiguan* and the *Sifeng* (Extra Points).

29. Pneumonia: *Neiguan*, Du 14 *Dazhui*, and Large Intestine 11 *Quchi*. Pneumonia is often a complication of the common cold. *Dazhui* raises the Yang and strengthens immunity. *Quchi* is famous for treating Heat.

30. Pleurisy: *Neiguan*, and Ren 17 *Shanzhong*.

31. Loss of voice due to Heat constrained by Cold ("Cold surrounds the Heat"): *Neiguan* plus Lung 10 *Yuji*. *Neiguan* opens the throat. *Yuji* is good for strengthening the voice and for voice loss.

32. Loss of voice caused by external Wind-Cold: *Neiguan*, Gall Bladder 20 *Fengchi*, Large Intestine 4 *Hegu*, and Lung 10 *Yuji*.

33. Loss of voice from lack of fluids caused by Yin *xu*: *Neiguan*, Lung 7 *Lieque*, Lung 10 *Yuji*, and Kidney 6 *Zhaohai*. Each of these points is very good for treating the throat.

34. Vomiting: *Neiguan*, Ren 22 *Tiantu*, and Stomach 36 *Zusanli*.

35. Vomiting: *Neiguan* plus Ren 13 *Shangwan*.

36. Nausea or vomiting: *Neiguan* alone.

37. **Hiccups:** *Neiguan* and Urinary Bladder 17 *Geshu*.

38. **Hiccups:** *Neiguan* alone. If chronic, add Ren 22 *Tiantu* and Ren 12 *Zhongwan*.

39. **Cholecystitis and cholelithiasis:** *Neiguan*, Urinary Bladder 19 *Danshu*, and Ren 12 *Zhongwan*. In modern times more practitioners use *Dannang* (Extra Point) instead of *Danshu*.

40. **Pain of indefinite origin** in the Heart, chest, or costal region: *Neiguan* and Pericardium 4 *Ximen*.

41. **Pain in the hypochondriac region:** *Neiguan* and Gall Bladder 34 *Yanglingquan*.

42. **Postoperative pain** after chest surgery: *Neiguan* alone.

43. **Pain or distention** of the chest, Stomach, or Stomach area: *Neiguan* plus Ren 12 *Zhongwan*.

44. **Pain** in the Stomach due to Cold and *qi* stagnation: *Neiguan* and Stomach 36 *Zusanli*, plus moxibustion on Ren 12 *Zhongwan*.

45. **Pain** in the Stomach and belching, due to weakness of the Spleen: *Neiguan*, Stomach 34 *Liangqiu*, and Spleen 4 *Gongsun*. If the pain is mild do not use Spleen 4.

46. **Upper abdominal pain:** *Neiguan* alone.

47. **Abdominal pain** induced by anger, unhappiness, or any strong emotion: *Neiguan*, plus Spleen 6 *Sanyinjiao*, and Liver 3 *Taichong*. For any kind of pain due to strong emotions, *Neiguan* alone can be used as preventative treatment.

48. **Pain before eating:** *Neiguan* and Spleen 6 *Sanyinjiao*.

49. **Pain after eating** which is not due to overeating: *Neiguan* plus Stomach 36 *Zusanli*.

50. **Stomach spasm:** *Neiguan* and Spleen 4 *Gongsun*. This prescription is also used for treating pain after a meal due to overeating.

51. **Leukorrhea:** *Neiguan* plus Ren 6 *Qihai*. These two points resolve the Damp discharge but do not fully treat the cause of the disease, so other points need to be added according to the diagnosis.

52. **Menstrual cramps:** *Neiguan* plus Spleen 6 *Sanyinjiao*. If pain is associated with Cold, then add moxibustion to Ren 4 *Guanyuan*.

53. **Infertility:** *Neiguan*, Ren 4 *Guanyuan*, and Kidney 7 *Fuliu*. Ren 6 *Qihai* may be added—or used alternately with Ren 4—in order to strengthen the patient's *qi*.

54. **Anemia:** *Neiguan*, Du 14 *Dazhui*, Urinary Bladder 18 *Ganshu*, and Spleen 6 *Sanyinjiao*. *Sanyinjiao* is an important point for any condition related to the blood.

55. **Heatstroke:** *Neiguan* and Pericardium 9 *Zhongchong*. Usually *Zhongchong* is bled for heatstroke or sunstroke. Most often the color of the blood is dark as it first exits the acupuncture point, so squeeze out small amounts of blood until the color is normal.

56. **Revival from drowning:** *Neiguan* with Ren 1 *Huiyin*, Du 25 *Suliao*, and Kidney 1 *Yongquan*. Ren 1 connects the Ren and the Du Channels. The needle insertion at *Huiyin* for this condition is very deep, up to 3 *cun*.

57. **Coma or shock:** *Neiguan*, *Renzhong* Du 26, and Stomach 36 *Zusanli*. When coma or shock is severe, the pulse is very deep and weak.

58. **Electrical shock:** *Neiguan*, Du 26 *Renzhong*, and Pericardium 9 *Zhongchong*. Originally, this formula was used for treating patients struck by lightning.

All of these *Neiguan* formulas are very effective and use only a few points. Prescriptions which use few points allow for the addition of acupuncture points to meet other needs which the patient may have.

6

Guidelines for Creating Prescriptions

Treatment with acupuncture is similar to treatment with Chinese herbs in that acupuncture points, like Chinese herbs, are combined to form a prescription according to a given problem. Finding a prescription to effect a cure or to alleviate a patient's suffering due to disease is by no means a mechanical process. Many factors contribute to the disease complex, and formulating an effective prescription for treatment comes from the insight gained through experience—both one's own experience and that garnered from other practitioners.

There are two distinct methods of arriving at prescriptions for treatment. One method is to utilize point combinations which have been established by historical precedent. Ancient Chinese culture remains a vital part of China's modern culture, unlike the cultures of ancient civilizations such as Egypt or the Near East; acupuncture's unique context is a cultural continuity spanning more than six millennia. The recorded experiences of more than three thousand years of medical practice have led to a large repertoire of acupuncture point combinations for treating many different problems.

The second method is to create point combinations. The ability to create an acupuncture prescription depends upon an understanding of how prescriptions are configured. It depends equally on a solid grasp of the specific therapeutic effects of approximately one hundred acupuncture points and their different effects when combined with one another. Skill at creating prescriptions also provides a means for altering established configurations of acupuncture points. This is similar to the way that Chinese herbalists add to and subtract from classical herbal prescriptions in order to tailor them to the unique needs of a patient.

Regardless of the manner in which a prescription is selected, it addresses three aspects of a disease condition: *Cause, Location,* and *Symptoms* (listed in order of importance).

Seven Forms of an Acupuncture Prescription

Acupuncture points are combined in seven ways. Selection of a specific form is based on the nature of the problem being treated.

Big Form

Big Form means that more needles than usual are used in a treatment, from ten to as many as fourteen needles. Needles used in Big Form are of bigger gauge and are retained for a longer time. In ancient times when needles were made of stone, prescriptions consisted of only one needle. As needles became more refined, the number of needles in a treatment increased, first to two needles, then to four, and later to as many as eight.

In most circumstances, the general rule of practice is to use as few needles as possible. Big Form is selected when treatment using only a few needles does not have a heavy enough effect to solve the problem. Conditions treated with the Big Form are severe. The effects of this form are heavy in the sense that there is greater therapeutic power or efficacy of treatment. Heavy should not be taken as synonymous with *xie* (Reducing). Big Form is not used often, and most definitely not for a patient who is receiving treatment for the first time.

Big Form has been used for infantile paralysis and for arthritis cases in which the pain is in many places. Customarily, treatment for children uses very few needles. Big Form is necessary for treatment of a problem as complex as infantile paralysis in order to get results. When treating children, however, the needle gauge is smaller and the strength of treatment is not as strong as for adults.

Many kinds of skin problems can be treated with a few needles rather than with the large number of needles in Big Form. Large Intestine 11 *Quchi* treats skin problems in the upper body, and Spleen 10 *Xuehai* treats skin problems in the lower body. Both Gall Bladder 31 *Fengshi* and *Sanyinjiao* Spleen 6 are used for skin problems that affect the whole body. Some chronic or intractable skin problems do not respond well to treatment even if all the aforementioned points are combined together in Big Form. In that case more points are added to the prescription, especially ones that help clean up the body via the digestive system. Possible points include Ren 10 *Xiawan*, Large Intestine 4 *Hegu*, Spleen 9 *Yinlingquan*, and Stomach 36 *Zusanli*. When a difficult skin condition also presents with itching, cupping the navel can help. The navel is a delicate area, so cups are taken off the navel every five minutes and then reapplied.

Big Form is used for severe problems such as heavy bleeding. If there is bleeding in the head area, many points are selected in the lower legs and feet. This follows the *Nei Jing* guidelines of selecting points in the lower body to treat conditions in the upper body. Points such as the *Xi* (Cleft) Points may be selected since they are very effective for treating bleeding. Moreover, when many points are placed in the lower extremities, *qi* is drawn downward away from the head. Since *qi* moves the blood, bringing *qi* away from the head to the lower body helps to stop the bleeding.

Treatment of bleeding is one example which shows that Big Form cannot be taken as synonymous with *xie* (Reducing). In this last example, the *qi* is drawn down to the lower extremities only by the heavier effect of Big Form. Even though *xie* techniques can reduce *qi* from the head, they are not applied in treatment of bleeding. Any application of *xie* (Reducing) will result in some reduction of *zhen qi* (the overall *qi* of the body). A patient who is bleeding suffers loss of blood and *yuan qi*, and any further reduction of *qi* would injure the patient. In addition, care should be taken to insure mild treatment for bleeding. Strong treatment induces more rapid *qi* flow which, in turn, could cause increased bleeding.

Small Form

Small Form uses few needles, uses finer gauge needles, and is lighter than Big Form. Light should not be taken to mean *bu* (Reinforcing). Small Form is used for different kinds of problems, and either *bu* or *xie* may be used with this prescriptive form in accordance with the diagnosis.

Usually this form is for treating acute problems. "Acute" in Chinese is literally "swift moving disease," and acute conditions generally respond quickly to treatment. Because acute problems can resolve quickly and more easily, the lighter therapy of Small Form is sufficient for effective treatment. Small Form is also selected for conditions, whether acute or not, that are light or not too severe, and for weak or delicate patients.

One particular patient is a good example of the variety of possible applications of the Small Form. This patient had very low resistance and was vulnerable to acute attacks of the common cold. What proved effective was the use of a single acupuncture point that could both relieve the surface of pathogenic factors and fortify the patient's resistance. Following the *Nei Jing's* advice that the Yangming Channel is one of the primary meridians for relieving the body surface of exterior pathogenic factors associated with the common cold, Stomach 36 *Zusanli* of the Foot-Yangming Channel was selected. First, *xie* technique was applied to *Zusanli* in order to relieve the surface. After applying *xie* technique a few times during the treatment, *bu* technique was applied during the latter portion of the treatment to strengthen the patient's resistance. Light application of moxibustion on *Zusanli* after the needle was removed helped emphasize the Reinforcing aspect of the treatment. In this one case, the application of Small Form included *xie* technique, *bu* technique, treatment of an acute condition, and treatment of a weak patient—all accomplished with only one needle.

Rapid Form

The Rapid Form is selected for treating urgent problems and emergencies. Points that are selected are expected to get results right away. Moreover, acupuncture points used in Rapid Form should be ones that can be quickly located and that have easier access for applying treatment than other points which could be selected for the same problem. Some examples are: moxibustion on the navel (Ren 8 *Shenque*) for unchecked diarrhea, Large Intestine 4 *Hegu* for severe headache, Ren 26 *Renzhong* for fainting, Stomach 36 *Zusanli* or Kidney 1 *Yongquan* for stroke, and Du 20 *Baihui* for seizures.

Slow Form

Slow Form uses few points, and needles are not retained for a long time. This form is applied to treatment of chronic problems, but ones which are not too serious. With chronic conditions there is Deficiency and lowered body function, so significant response to treatment is not expected right away. The frequency of treatment corresponds with the expected rate of recovery, which is gradual or "slow."

Generally, the preferred therapeutic style in China is treating daily or every other day. However, Slow Form begins with treatment only twice a week, is reduced to once a week after continual signs of recovery, and is later reduced to once every two weeks. Examples of mild chronic problems that can be treated with the Slow Form are constipation, nervousness, insomnia, and memory loss.

A common type of chronic constipation among the elderly occurs as a result of dryness. With aging comes a gradual Deficiency of *qi,* and the ensuing dryness is a consequence of the lowered body function that corresponds with Deficiency. A simple and effective prescription from the *Zhen Jiu Da Cheng* by Yang Ji-Zhou uses only Spleen 14 *Fujie* on the left side of the body to treat this kind of constipation. First, *bu* technique is applied to fortify the patient and promote moisture. Then, light *xie* technique is administered in order to induce movement of the bowel. *Fujie* is selected on the left side of the body because it is located over the descending colon.

Odd Form

Also known as the Single Form, the Odd Form uses only one acupuncture point. In cases of pain that affects both sides of the body, the point is needled bilaterally. Bilateral needling is also applied when problems are severe, in order to amplify the effects of the treatment.

Following are a few Odd Form prescriptions:

Seizures: Ren 17 *Shanzhong*. In ancient times Liver 3 *Taichong* was often used. Another point that has come into favor in modern times is Ren 15 *Jiuwei*.

Dizziness: Large Intestine 4 *Hegu*, now considered a master point for the head. A prescription for dizziness from ancient times is Du 20 *Baihui*.

Insomnia resulting from anger or any strong emotion: Liver 2 *Xingjian*.

Poor digestion: Ren 12 *Zhongwan*. Modern prescriptions add Ren 6 *Qihai* to move the *qi* and thus aid the digestion, and also add Stomach 36 *Zusanli* and Spleen 6 *Sanyinjiao*.

Low back pain due to straining while lifting: Urinary Bladder 40 *Weizhong*. If the pain also radiates down the leg and *Weizhong* is not effective enough, then Gall Bladder 30 *Huantiao* is used instead. *Huantiao* is a good point for treating problems that link the torso and the legs.

Low back pain due to weakness or to Kidney *xu:* Either Urinary Bladder 23 *Shenshu* or Kidney 3 *Taixi*.

When diagnosis provides certainty as to the cause, one point can be enough to treat the problem.

Even Form

A description of this form is that points are "always paired." The number of needles inserted on the left side of the body is matched by an equal number of points on the right side. This does not necessarily mean that the same point is needled bilaterally. Though the number of points on each side of the body is the same, the specific points that are selected may vary from side to side.

Even Form is used for treating problems that affect the whole body, problems like general weakness or lowered resistance to the common cold, flu, or other exterior pathogenic factors. No matter what the other therapeutic properties of a specific prescription, the use of Even Form treats and balances the whole body, an effect achieved simply by placing points in even numbers on both sides of the body.

The Four Gates (Large Intestine 4 *Hegu* and Liver 3 *Taichong*) is one effective prescription for dispelling outside pathogenic factors as well as for promoting the body's general resistance to exterior factors. All four points may be selected, or just one point can be inserted on each side. With only two needles—one *Hegu* on one side of the body and one *Taichong* on the other side—the prescriptive effect of the Four Gates plus the added effect of Even Form can be obtained.

Inserting points in even numbers on the front and back of the body at the same time can also constitute Even Form, such as when needling Urinary Bladder 13 *Feishu* and Lung 1 *Zhongfu* to treat asthma. Simultaneously needling these points is accomplished by having the patient sit up for treatment rather than recline. Special attention should be given to inserting needles at *Zhongfu;* if the Lung is touched when needling Lung 1, a pneumothorax may occur. Therefore, inserting a needle obliquely toward the shoulder can prevent the occurrence of this problem. This prescription of *Feishu* plus *Zhongfu* is one variation of Yin-Yang therapy, which in this case uses both the Back-*Shu* and the Front-*Mu* Points at the same time.

Another prescription, Du 14 *Dazhui* plus Ren 4 *Guanyuan*, is also known as Yin-Yang therapy because it reinforces the Yin and Yang of the whole body. Needles can be retained in both these points at the same time by having the patient sit for treatment. Or, if the needle at *Dazhui* is inserted horizontally downward, the patient can lie down after the needle is inserted at Du 14 and a needle can then be placed in *Guanyuan*. To enhance the effects of this treatment, one needle can be placed at Stomach 36 *Zusanli* and another can be inserted on the other side at Spleen 6 *Sanyinjiao*. In spite of adding these latter two needles to this variation of Yin-Yang therapy, one on the left and one on the right, this prescription is still considered Even Form.

The general effect provided by Even Form is important for treating trauma. The impulse of trauma damages the flow of the *sanjiao qi* (*qi* of the whole body). Damage to the smooth flow of the *sanjiao qi* can manifest in ways such as loss of energy or general weakness, headaches, and body ache. Impaired flow of the *sanjiao qi* due to trauma can also induce insomnia, diminished mental clarity, or mood swings. Due to the effects of trauma on the whole body *qi*, any or all of these symptoms can come and go, at times seemingly without reason for their appearance. A prescription that can quickly meet the acute needs of trauma is most effective with the general balancing added by Even Form.

Complex Form

Complex Form is for treating complex problems. One meaning of complex is that a condition is difficult to treat. If a prescription does not seem to have strong enough effect, points are added which have effects similar to those already being used. Additional points that are chosen need not be from the same meridians already selected. For example, high blood pressure which causes headache or stiff neck can be treated with Gall Bladder 20 *Fengchi*, which is an effective point for treating stiff neck, headache, or high blood pressure, whether these symptoms appear together or not. If the symptoms are severe, *Fengchi* is needled bilaterally. Usually, needling Gall Bladder 20 alone will cause the blood pressure to drop and make the headache go away. If the treatment is not effective, Urinary Bladder 10 *Tianzhu* can be added to the prescription to amplify its effects.

Complex can also mean that a patient presents with more than one health problem at the same time. Diagnosis of the different complaints determines whether or not a point prescription can be formulated to treat the different conditions simultaneously. If not, they must be dealt with through separate courses of treatment.

Two variations of the Complex Form treat different problems simultaneously: the Duplicate Complex Form and the Separate Complex Form. In the Duplicate variety, a point which can treat both problems is added. One example is a patient with arthritic knee pain who, at the time of treatment, also complained of acute stomachache. The prescription first consisted of Ren 12 *Zhongwan* for the Stomach pain and *Xiyan* (Extra Points) for the arthritic pain. After a short time of treatment there was little change in the stomachache. Stomach 36 *Zusanli* was then added because of its ability to treat both the Stomach and the knee pain.

Treatment of post-stroke paralysis can be complex because stroke patients present with many problems at the same time. Both the meridians and the internal organs can be affected. Emotional issues may have preceded the stroke but will certainly come about due to the paralysis. Often with stroke conditions there is a mixture of Excess, Deficiency, Hot, Cold, and phlegm. A practitioner who does well at treating stroke can also be successful at treating a wide range of other problems.

So, when forming prescriptions for treatment of stroke, it is important to be able to add points to the prescription that treat more than one aspect of the stroke at the same time. Du 16 *Fengfu* is an important point for treating loss of voice, blurring of vision, and high blood pressure. In addition, it helps treat paralysis of the lower extremities. Large Intestine 11 *Quchi* is one of the main points for treating paralysis of the arm. Many post-stroke patients develop constipation and *Quchi* is also a good point for regulating the bowel. Stroke patients may experience significant decrease in appetite. A point which increases the appetite and also treats paralysis of the arm is Large Intestine 10 *Shousanli*. Stomach 36 *Zusanli* is an important emergency point for stroke because of its ability to readjust the vital function of the internal organs. *Zusanli* is used post-stroke as a tonic point to Reinforce the patient's *qi*, to treat paralysis of the legs, to increase the appetite and digestive functions, and to eliminate phlegm. Moxibustion on *Zusanli* and Gall Bladder 39 *Xuanzhong* is an important prophylactic for stroke. After a stroke, if there are signs that another stroke is possible, direct moxibustion is applied to *Zusanli* and *Xuanzhong* twice daily.

When stroke causes paralysis of the upper and lower body and there is also speech impairment, prescriptions may seem to be Big Form because of the larger number of needles used in each treatment. However, there are some differences from the Big Form. Stroke patients suffer damage to *qi* and blood and, because of their weakness, often cannot tolerate strong treatment. For that reason, it is possible with patients who are weak and very sensitive to treatment to remove most—if not all—needles right after needling sensation *(de qi)* is achieved. This approach prevents the treatment from being too strong for the patient. In contrast, in Big Form, needles are retained for a long time. Also, when this lighter approach is taken with stroke patients, smaller gauge needles are used. In contrast, the Big Form uses larger gauge needles.

The Separate Complex Form is also for treating more than one problem at a time, but it adds points which treat each problem separately. One example is a patient who was being treated for facial paralysis due to Bell's Palsy. The basic prescription was one needle on the affected side from Stomach 4 *Dicang* to Stomach 6 *Jiache* (Through and Through Puncturing), and one needle at Large Intestine 4 *Hegu* on the opposite side. During the course of treatment the patient developed an acute case of urticaria. Large Intestine 11 *Quchi* and Large Intestine 14 *Binao* were added to the prescription to treat the urticaria even though these two points had no effect on the facial paralysis. It was possible to treat both conditions simultaneously because the basic prescription was small and allowed for the addition of points even though they did not treat the original problem. If this had not been possible, treatment of the acute problem would have taken precedence over treatment of the facial paralysis because of the urgency of the urticaria, and because the original problem was not one which would resolve in a short time.

The Ten Agents of Acupuncture Prescriptions

The ten agents of acupuncture point prescriptions are classifications of prescriptions according to their therapeutic effects, the manner in which combinations of points function.

Reinforcing

From a treatment point of view, great emphasis is placed not only on fortifying a weakened body and building a strong constitution when there is disease, but also on promoting continued good health and well-being when there is absence of disease.

The most famous point for Reinforcing the Yang is Du 14 *Dazhui*. An acupuncture point that is often combined with *Dazhui* for treating Yang *xu*, for regulating the Yang, and for strengthening the back, is Du 13 *Taodao*. "*Taodao*" means "to make excited," and the effects of Du 14 are amplified ("excited") when combined with *Taodao*. When these two points are used together, not only are the effects of *Dazhui* more powerful, the therapeutic response tends to be quicker.

Moxibustion on any one of three points—Urinary Bladder 43 *Gaohuangshu*, Gall Bladder 39 *Xuanzhong*, and Stomach 36 *Zusanli*—fortifies the whole body. *Gaohuangshu* is an important point to Reinforce the Lung, to treat pulmonary tuberculosis, and to lift resistance. *Xuanzhong* is very effective for raising immunity, and moxibustion on this point has a positive effect on T cell production. *Zusanli* may well be the single most important acupuncture point for applying moxibustion to obtain a wide range of effects.

Retroaction

The effect of Retroaction is to alter or counteract abnormal flow of *qi*. Nausea, vomiting, or hiccupping occur when *qi* rises rather than descends as it normally should. *Neiguan* Pericardium 6 is usually the first point selected for treating nausea, vomiting, and hiccupping. Ren 17 *Shanzhong*, the Influential Point for *qi*, may be combined with *Neiguan* because these problems are related to *qi*.

High blood pressure is an abnormal rising of *qi*. The causes of high blood pressure are many and complex. A number of prescriptions help to bring the *qi* down and quickly lower the blood pressure, but these prescriptions do not necessarily address the variety of underlying causes which must also be diagnosed and treated in each case. One prescription to lower blood pressure is the combination of *Neiguan* and *Zusanli*. This small and simple prescription allows room for the insertion of other needles to treat the underlying cause. A needle placed in *Zusanli* on the right side of the body is more effective for pulling the *qi* downward, since the right side is the *qi* side of the body (evidenced by radial pulses on the right side that are associated with *qi*: the Lung, the Spleen, and the Kidney Yang or *Mingmen*).

Moxibustion or needles applied to *Zusanli* on the right side are used to pull the *qi* downward and help the Kidneys grasp the *qi* in cases of dyspnea or shortness of breath.

Light

"Light" means the use of mild stimulation for Excess conditions. Liver Fire and Excess Liver Yang are disturbances of the Liver with Excess symptoms such as red eyes, irritability, red face, dizziness, headache, and high blood pressure. Patients with such symptoms may suffer from a stroke at any time, and inappropriately strong needle stimulation can actually induce a stroke. An effective prescription for treating these conditions is mild stimulation of Urinary Bladder 17 *Geshu*. Since these symptoms are severe ones, a way to amplify the effects of the treatment without using strong stimulation is to needle *Geshu* bilaterally.

Two acupuncture points used for these same symptoms are Du 16 *Fengfu* and Stomach 9 *Renying*. Because of the position of *Fengfu* over the spine and near the brain, it is a delicate and potentially dangerous point. The stimulus of *Fengfu* tends to be very strong as well. *Renying* is most effective for treating these Excess conditions if the needle insertion is deep. The use of either *Fengfu* or *Renying* is not as safe as mild stimulation of *Geshu*. Another means of bringing down the blood pressure is (starting at *Geshu*) repeated insertion and withdrawal of a needle downward along the Urinary Bladder Channel using mild stimulation. This lightly encourages the *qi* to descend.

Constipation is an Excess that may appear in patients who are Deficient, such as the elderly. The constipation is a localized Excess, but the underlying cause is one of Deficiency. In such cases, the best way to eliminate the Excess accumulation in the bowel is mild or light treatment. According to classical texts, commonly used points for constipation are Sanjiao 6 *Zhigou* and Ren 6 *Qihai*. Substitute points for this combination are bilateral insertion at Stomach 25 *Tianshu* or at Spleen 15 *Daheng*.

Ventilation

The meaning of Ventilation is to "to make smooth," "to mobilize," or "to circulate," and it is used to remove stagnation. Stomach 40 *Fenglong* is a point famous for treating stagnated phlegm, though usually *Fenglong* is not effective enough when used by itself. For phlegm stagnated in the throat, *Fenglong* is combined with Ren 22 *Tiantu*. *Tiantu* is used not only for phlegm but also for stubborn cough, traditionally attributed to *qi* stagnation. Wheezing is a sign of stagnated phlegm, and a prescription for treating bronchial wheezing includes Pericardium 6 *Neiguan*, Stomach 40 *Fenglong*, and Liver 2 *Xingjian*. Points may be added that promote smooth flow of *qi*, such as *Tiantu* and *Zusanli*.

Purgation

Purgation is used to open up stagnation (*zhi*—literally, "stiffness"). Stiffness means that something stays or is stuck. The dispersing effects of Purgation permit unobstructed flow of *qi* and eliminate stagnation.

Dysentery presents with pus and blood in the stool, and tenesmus. Tenesmus is an uncomfortable sensation due to stagnation and it indicates that, in spite of frequent bowel movement, pathogens are stuck inside. A point prescription for dysentery is Ren 5 *Shimen* plus Stomach 25 *Tianshu*. For acute cases, treatment from one to three times daily can effectively treat dysentery within two to three days. *Shimen* is contraindicated for young women; due to its close proximity to the uterus, needling *Shimen* can cause sterility. Points which may be used as substitutes for *Shimen* are Ren 12 *Zhongwan*, Ren 6 *Qihai*, and Stomach 36 *Zusanli*.

Astringent

The Astringent agent of an acupuncture prescription treats prolapse, the slipping of organs from their proper position.

Prolapse of the rectum is treated with Du 20 *Baihui,* plus Du 1 *Changqiang* as a local point. A pair of points also used for rectal prolapse is *Erbai* (Extra Points), located 4 *cun* proximal to Pericardium 7 *Daling.*

Primary points for treating prolapse of the uterus are Gall Bladder 28 *Weidao,* Kidney 3 *Taixi,* and Liver 3 *Taichong.* This point combination is also used for treatment of Kidney prolapse.

Prolapse occurs due to Deficiency. Kidney 3 *Taixi* is an important point for treating Deficiency and is considered one of the best points to include in any prescription for treatment of prolapse.

Lubrication

The effect of Lubrication is to discharge any abnormal concretion. Like Ventilation, the meaning of Lubrication is "to make smooth." In the case of Lubrication, stagnation is relieved by bringing out fluid.

To remove ganglia, the ganglia is palpated to determine its root. Four needles are inserted around the ganglia ninety degrees apart from each other and under its root area. After the needles are removed, the ganglia is pressed to remove fluid.

Pricking or slicing the *Sifeng* (Extra Points) and squeezing out a small amount of yellowish viscous fluid is indicated for treating malnutrition and indigestion in young children. If the *Sifeng* bleed from being pricked or sliced, the treatment is not effective. Digestive problems are common in children and indicate concretion of the *zhong qi* (Central *qi*). The *zhong qi* is the functions of the Middle *jiao*—meaning the Stomach and the Spleen—in digesting and transporting nutrients. Concretion of the Central *qi* is a congealing of *qi* due to poor circulation, poor *qi* activity. Children's digestive problems are typically due to weakness of the digestive system, and Lubrication in this instance should not be taken to mean *xie* (Reducing) technique in order "to make smooth" the functioning of the *zhong qi*.

Sedation

Sedation is used for occlusion or closed cases. Occlusion is extreme stagnation, and is considered more severe than *shi* (Excess).

The agent of Sedation must not be taken to simply mean *xie* (Reducing), for some cases of occlusion are caused by Deficiency. One such example is retention of urine among the elderly. The urinary flow is blocked due to a weakness of *qi*. Treatment for urine retention among the elderly includes moxibustion over the whole lower abdomen, plus needles inserted into Urinary Bladder 53 *Baohuang* and Urinary Bladder 54 *Zhibian*. The use of moxa warms the Lower *jiao* and helps to open the blockage by both mildly fortifying and circulating the *qi*.

Severe constipation due to Excess heat, stagnated food, or *qi* Deficiency may be treated using only Kidney 18 *Shiquan*. Diagnosis determines which technique is appropriate to apply to *Shiquan* for the different causes of constipation. Yang Ji-Zhou used only Spleen 6 *Sanyinjiao* for treating severe constipation. The fact that some of his contemporaries were unable to obtain results using Spleen 6 alone is a testimony to Yang Ji-Zhou's high level of skill.

Moisturizing Overcomes Dryness

Common signs of Dryness are thirst, dry skin, and itching. The treatment principle is to Reinforce the *qi* (vital function) in order to produce more blood and cultivate more body fluid. A prescription that matches this principle of treatment uses Urinary Bladder 17 *Geshu*, Ren 17 *Shanzhong*, and Kidney 3 *Taixi*. *Shanzhong* is the point for *qi*, *Geshu* for blood; *Taixi* is one of the most important points for promoting fluid.

According to Chinese medicine, hysteria occurs when fluids are dry and *qi* is Deficient. Blood Deficiency caused by the *qi* Deficiency (lowered vital function) turns to Heat and results in hysteria. A prescription for treating the symptoms of hysteria—Ren 14 *Juque*, Pericardium 6 *Neiguan*, and Heart 7 *Shenmen*—can be combined with points from the prescription above for Dryness. Patients suffering from hysteria should avoid intake of foods that produce Heat: greasy or oily food, spicy food, meat, chocolate, and coffee.

When symptoms of Dryness and Heat appear together, first *xie* (Reduce) the heat and then *bu* (Reinforce) the fluids. The general practice is to apply some *xie* technique at the beginning of treatment to first eliminate the presence of any pathogenic factors (*xie qi*, "Evil *qi*"). Beginning a treatment with *bu* technique can inhibit the elimination of pathogens. Large Intestine 11 *Quchi* and Large Intestine 4 *Hegu* eliminate Heat from the upper body, and Spleen 10 *Xuehai* eliminates Heat from the lower body. Either Kidney 3 *Taixi* or Spleen 6 *Sanyinjiao* may be used to promote fluids.

Drying Overcomes Moisture
Problems with moisture can be traced to the Spleen, Stomach, and Kidney. Some signs of moisture are pitting edema, eczema, urine retention, and swelling such as non-pitting edema. Chinese medicine also views flatulence and a sense of fullness in the Stomach without having eaten as signs of moisture associated with *non-vaporization of qi*. Non-vaporization of *qi*

means that poor circulation of *qi* causes a condensation of *qi* and fluids at a subtle level.

He-Sea Points of the Stomach and Spleen are often selected for overcoming problems with moisture. For severe conditions, Spleen 3 *Taibai* and Kidney 5 *Shuiquan* are added to prescriptions. *Taibai* strengthens the functions of the Spleen and Stomach to control moisture. *Shuiquan* opens meridian blockage and raises activity of the Kidney Yang to clean up pathogenic moisture.

The agent of Drying to Overcome Moisture is directed at treating the whole body. An understanding of the way the symptoms are linked with the underlying cause provides a window to the whole system involved.

PART III

ACUPUNCTURE TECHNIQUES

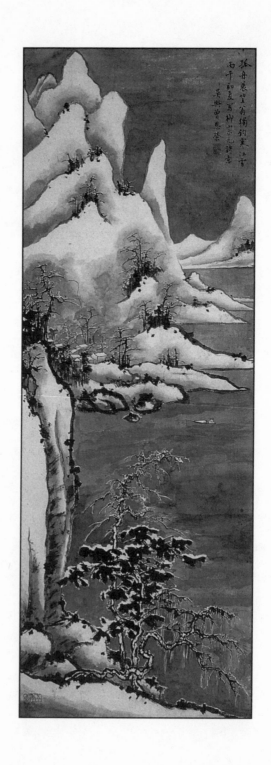

"Before you put your hands on any patient,
stop, say a prayer, and remember:
it's not you that is doing the healing."

Mrs. Tseng-Ni Qian Yun
(A mother's advice to her son at
the beginning of his medical career)

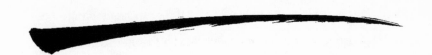

7

Classical Needling Techniques

The Historical Use of Needles and the Development of Techniques

Within the *Nei Jing* are so many different acupuncture techniques that the information is overwhelming. The text yields too many needling techniques to easily keep in mind; some of the techniques even have seemingly contradictory effects, leading to confusion for some practitioners.

Over the centuries, traditional practitioners have chosen to employ certain classical techniques over others. Most notable are the Five Ancient Insertion Methods associated with pathological changes of the five *zang* organs, the Nine Ancient Insertion Methods based on uses of the Nine Ancient Needles, and the Twelve Ancient Methods of Insertion into the Twelve Regular Channels.

Over time, ways of applying these techniques evolved, with changes in the type of needles being used as well as entirely different ways of administering some of the techniques. In addition, due to the therapeutic effects these techniques can provide, use of these various needling methods has expanded into areas of treatment different from their original uses. We can find evidence of this in books by the most influential physicians throughout China's history. By drawing on examples from such a wealth of experience, we can acquire an ample variety of techniques well proven to provide the most effective treatment.

Archaeological evidence shows that acupuncture dates back to China's Neolithic times, and that the first known acupuncture needles were made from stone: one needle for scraping the skin to stimulate the meridians, one for lancing superficial abscesses, and one for insertion. Because the needle for insertion was so crude, treatments originally consisted of inserting only one needle, and ancient practitioners were challenged to select the best possible point for any given treatment. Moreover, many different effects had to be obtained from a single needle, and meeting this need led to developments of acupuncture techniques as well as to further refinements of acupuncture needles.

The use of stone acupuncture needles for insertion, called *bian*, first appeared in northern China. Generally, the body type of northern Chinese is more robust and muscular than that of southern Chinese. This led to a needling style in the north that is deeper than in southern China, and acupuncturists in northern China have historically made more varied use of acupuncture techniques. The cold northern climate also promoted the development of moxa therapy, and, as can be expected, use of moxibustion has prevailed among northern practitioners. From ancient times to the present, the acupuncture style in northern China has tended toward deeper needling and stronger techniques than that in the south, as well as the use of more moxibustion.

Coastal areas of China first used fish bone and animal bone for acupuncture needles. Another material in early use was very hard wood. Copper was one of the first metal needles, selected for its ability to conduct heat. The practice of warming the handle of a needle to transmit heat into acupuncture points is an ancient technique. Iron, gold, and silver all came into use as materials for acupuncture needles. Gold and silver were used for pain relief. Because both silver and gold are too soft, red copper was blended with them for a firmer needle.

Currently, the stainless steel filiform needle is the most frequently used, and great emphasis is placed on its manipulation. A good quality needle has a round and smooth body, a tip that is not too sharp or too dull, and flexibility and strength. A filiform needle is very fine and flexible, so it demands precise finger force from the practitioner. In return, the filiform needle can provide precise manipulations that make it very effective for performing a wide variety of techniques. Prior to refinements leading to the design of the modern filiform needle in the 2nd century AD, clinical needles were still based on the Nine Ancient Needles, with the performance of different techniques made possible, in part, by the variety of needle being used.

Theoretical and technological developments of Chinese medicine have occurred gradually. Medical theories and clinical experiences have been compiled from many disparate sources since the practice of medicine in China has been segmented regionally, with more emphasis on herbs in the south and more emphasis on acupuncture and moxibustion in the north. Regional differences also led to different treatment styles, such as the shallow insertion of needles typical among practitioners in the hot southern climates. Some northern practitioners even practice moxibustion to the exclusion of all other modes of therapy.

The Tang Dynasty of one thousand years ago is known for the high level of skill of many of its physicians. Yet during that time, seldom did a physician practice both herbal therapy and acupuncture. Many of the Tang Dynasty acupuncturists never used moxibustion, only needles. To this day it is common to find practitioners who practice mostly one aspect of traditional Chinese medicine rather than a broad scope of medicine based equally on acupuncture, Chinese herbs, moxibustion, diet, health exercises, and therapeutic massage.

One of the most notable physicians to practice all aspects of Chinese medicine was the great Hua Tuo, who was executed while in his late nineties around AD 200. Some people attribute refinements of the modern filiform needle to Hua Tuo. Even if Hua Tuo is not actually responsible for development of the modern needle, he is the foremost practitioner to take advantage of the significant refinements of acupuncture needles that occurred in his lifetime. He is the first known practitioner to insert needles into points previously considered too dangerous to needle, such as Urinary Bladder 43 *Gaohuangshu* and Du 17 *Naohu*. Hua Tuo is the first known doctor to prescribe health exercises and hydrotherapy. He was an acupuncturist, herbalist, and surgeon, but because of Hua Tuo's skill as an acupuncturist and his discovery of the Hua Tuo Jiaji Points, he is mostly thought of as an acupuncturist. Few think of his skill as a surgeon and as an outstanding herbalist who developed herbal anesthesia for surgery. For political reasons, many of Hua Tuo's writings were destroyed shortly after his death. A scholar-physician named Ge Hong, born 80 years after Hua Tuo's death, collected, compiled, and disseminated writings by Hua Tuo.

Li Dong-Yuan lived about 1,000 years after Hua Tuo. He is best known as an herbalist because of his masterpiece, *Treatise on the Spleen and Stomach.* So important are his contributions as an herbalist that he usually is not recognized as a highly skilled acupuncturist. An equally great contribution by Li Dong-Yuan is his research leading to the revival of a *Nei Jing* acupuncture technique, *Dao Qi.*

Li Shi-Zhen is another physician who excelled at different aspects of Chinese medicine. The contributions from his book *Ben Cao Gang Mu (Compendium of Materia Medica),* published four hundred years ago, rank him as one of the foremost herbalists in all of Chinese history. This book consists of fifty-two volumes and took over thirty years to compile. The *Ben Cao Gang Mu,* more than a pharmaceutical compendium, goes into natural sciences that include botany, zoology, mineralogy, and metallurgy. It contains listings of nearly 1,900 medical substances, with detailed descriptions of the appearance, method of collection, preparation, and use of each substance. It contains more than 1,000 illustrations and over 10,000 prescriptions. Even more remarkable is that this is only one of a dozen books written by Li Shi-Zhen. His work, *The Pulse Studies of Bin Hu,* is one of the standards for pulse diagnosis. In spite of his accomplishments, Li Shi-Zhen is seldom recognized as an outstanding acupuncturist even though his work, *A Study of the Eight Extra Channels,* is one of the most important books for acupuncturists on this subject.

Refinements in the subtlety, nuance, and effectiveness of acupuncture treatment came with refinements in the quality of needles. As needles became less crude, the number of needles used in a treatment increased, which promoted more sophisticated configuration of point prescriptions and allowed treatment of more complex conditions. In addition, advancements in the quality of needles promoted developments in higher levels of technical skill. Throughout history, the classical style of acupuncture has undergone developments while it has maintained the influences of ancient times, with continued emphasis both on the use of as few needles as possible in a treatment and on the application of acupuncture techniques for efficacy of treatment.

Chart 7-1.

TWELVE ANCIENT METHODS OF INSERTION INTO THE TWELVE REGULAR CHANNELS

Ou Ci	Even Puncturing
Bao Ci	Trail Puncturing
Hui Ci	Relaxing Puncturing
Qi Ci	Team Puncturing
Yang Ci	Light Puncturing
Zhi Ci	Straight In Puncturing
Shu Ci	Transport Puncturing
Duan Ci	Short Puncturing
Fu Ci	Floating Puncturing
Yin Ci	Yin Puncturing
Bang Ci	Strengthen Puncturing
Zan Ci	Assistant Puncturing

Chart 7-2.

NINE ANCIENT INSERTION METHODS
BASED ON USES OF THE NINE ANCIENT NEEDLES

Shu Ci	*Shu* Point Puncturing
Yuan Dao Ci	Remote Puncturing
Jing Ci	Channel Puncturing
Luo Ci	Collateral Puncturing
Fen Ci	Divide Puncturing
Da Xie Ci	Heavy Puncturing
Mao Ci	Hair Puncturing
Ju Ci	Giant Puncturing
Cui Ci	Flame Needle Puncturing

Chart 7-3.

FIVE ANCIENT INSERTION METHODS
BASED ON PATHOLOGICAL CHANGES OF
THE FIVE *ZANG* ORGANS

Ban Ci (Lung)	Half Puncturing
Bao Wen Ci (Heart)	Leopard Puncturing
Guan Ci (Liver)	Joint Puncturing
He Gu Ci (Spleen)	Valley Puncturing
Shu Gu Ci (Kidney)	Bone Puncturing

Six Types of Insertion According to the *Nei Jing*

I. Superficial Puncturing

Of all the different groups of acupuncture techniques this is the most shallow, with insertion depth ranging from the skin's surface to just a little under the skin.

Hair *(Mao Ci)*

This is one of the Nine Ancient Insertion Methods based on uses of the Nine Ancient Needles. The word *"Mao"* ("hair") indicates insertion that is very shallow. Originally, *Mao Ci* was superficial puncturing of the skin with a short filiform needle to treat hypoesthesia and numbness of the skin due to poor circulation and Cold.

Hair Puncturing now includes the therapy of light tapping on the surface of the skin with a Cutaneous Needle. Cutaneous Needles are unique, best described as a type of hammer from which only the tips of a number of needles protrude. Three varieties of Cutaneous Needles are: the Plum Blossom Needle with 5 needles, the Seven Star Needle with 7 needles, and the Luo Han Needle with 18 needles. The more needles there are in the head of a Cutaneous Needle, the finer the gauge of the needle tips and the lighter the stimulus of tapping.

Stimulus is provided by continual light tapping of the affected area or desired acupuncture point. The Cutaneous Needle is held at the end of its handle between the thumb and index finger. Grasping the needle this way provides the hammering movement with more flexibility and can make the tapping seem to happen on its own. Regardless of the strength of treatment, the rate and the strength of tapping should be even in order to prevent inadvertent damage to the skin. A practitioner who has control over the evenness and the strength of Cutaneous hammering can treat a wide range of problems, based on the points selected and the strength of tapping on the points.

When treating skin problems such as herpes zoster or eczema, the skin is hammered until small red dots (petechiae) begin to appear. Then the area is cupped to cause light bleeding to help remove pathogenic Heat.

One current style of treatment for hypoesthesia or numbness of the skin utilizes a Cutaneous Needle rather than a filiform needle. Stimulation is along meridians in the affected areas as well as on any remaining areas with symptoms. The skin is tapped until a slight flush shows increased signs of circulation, but never to the point that any bleeding occurs. Applying moxibustion over the affected area immediately after the cutaneous tapping increases the therapeutic response to treatment.

Light tapping with the Cutaneous Needle is also used for delicate patients and for patients who are fearful of needles. A practitioner can, with very light hammering, obtain therapeutic effects from points and do so within the patient's range of comfort. Weak patients who have a headache may be treated by tapping from the first lumbar vertebra down to the fourth sacral vertebra, either on the Du Channel or on the Hua Tuo Jiaji Points; tapping on the local area of head pain and where the affected channels run through the area of pain is combined with hammering on the low back if the patient can tolerate the strength of treatment. Tapping Stomach 36 *Zusanli* and applying light moxibustion afterward treats morning sickness or poor appetite during pregnancy. Cutaneous tapping on Lung 7 *Lieque* may be used to treat young children with cough.

Half Puncturing *(Ban Ci)*

Ban Ci is one of the Five Ancient Insertion Methods used in accordance with pathological changes of the five *zang* organs. Half Puncturing is associated with the Lung, and was first used in ancient times for treatment of pulmonary tuberculosis. The Lung is also associated with the skin and with body hair. Because of its shallow depth of insertion, Half Puncturing may be used to treat skin problems.

Either a half-*cun* or one-*cun* filiform needle is the typical needle used for Half Puncturing. The strength of insertion is as light as possible, and needles are withdrawn as soon as *qi* arrives *(de qi)*. Though sometimes the sensation of this kind of insertion and withdrawal feels like a hair being pulled, the stimulus of *Ban Ci* should be kept light.

The superficial insertion and the light stimulus of *Ban Ci* make it appropriate for treating young children aged one month old to eight years old, and for treating delicate patients. The mild stimulus of *Ban Ci* also makes it suitable for treating bleeding. Treatment to stop bleeding should be mild, since strong treatment can accelerate the flow of *qi* and thereby increase blood flow.

Floating *(Fu Ci)*

"Floating" means that needles are inserted only at the outermost level. Floating Puncturing may be perpendicular, horizontal, or oblique, but it always is just beneath the surface of the skin and no deeper than the surface of the muscle.

Insertion at Lung 7 *Lieque* is horizontally upward, accomplished by pinching up the skin while inserting the needle just beneath the skin. The

longer the needle insertion at *Lieque* is up the forearm, the more effective
it is for treating cough.

Fu Ci may also be used for treatment of muscle spasm due to
superficial Cold and poor circulation. Cold conditions often call for
deeper needling, but when a condition is still at a superficial level the
corresponding depth of insertion is shallow.

Needles may be retained for a few hours, or for days. Treatment
using ear points may be with half-*cun* filiform needles that are retained no
longer than the length of an office visit. Or, Interdermal needles may be
retained in the ear from several days up to one week. There are two kinds
of Interdermal needles. The thumbtack Interdermal needle is the type
inserted in ear points. The grain-like type of Interdermal needle, about
one centimeter long with a head like a grain of wheat, is for insertion
in body points like Lung 7 for treating chronic cough. Interdermal
needles imbedded for days at a time are frequently used to treat chronic
and persistent painful diseases.

Fu Ci is one of the Twelve Ancient Methods of Insertion into the
Twelve Regular Channels.

Straight In *(Zhi Ci)*

Of all the Superficial types of insertion, *Zhi Ci* goes in the deepest, though
the insertion depth is still close to the surface of the body.

For the past several hundred years, some practitioners have taken
the meaning of Straight *(Zhi)* as synonymous with perpendicular insertion.
The ancient meaning of *"Zhi"* is "straight in" or "going straight in," that
is, inserting directly to the desired depth of needling without first waiting
for the *qi* to arrive.

Use of *Zhi Ci* was originally for treatment of superficial muscle spasm. When superficial muscle layers are pinched up with the pressing hand, it is easy to detect muscle that is in spasm and insert a needle directly into it. Pinching up muscle with the pressing hand during insertion not only aids going directly to the desired depth in the muscle, it also prevents damage to the muscle from insertion that is too deep. Pinching up in this manner is also helpful if the needle insertion is on the torso since it prevents inadvertent insertion into the body cavity.

The concept of Straight In, going directly to the desired depth, is an important technique for treating febrile conditions. When there is fever, insertion should be shallow, going quickly to the desired depth. Inserting too deeply causes pathogenic factors ("Evil *qi*," *xie qi*) to penetrate, and insertion that is slow draws the Evil *qi* inward. Arrival of *qi* (needling reaction) and *xie* (Reducing) of pathogenic factors need to be accomplished at a superficial level when there is fever.

Straight In is also applied for itching and urticaria, problems that have superficial locations and also have pathogenic Heat. Levels of insertion, such as Superficial Puncturing and Deep Puncturing, differ according to the level of the disorder. Ideally the needle should go to the area or to the level that is affected.

Zhi Ci is one of the Twelve Ancient Methods of Insertion.

II. Deep Puncturing

Deep Puncturing is for problems deep in muscle, in the joint, close to the bone, or in the bone. Insertion using Deep Puncturing for problems deep in tissue, such as muscle or tendon, may be only a little deeper than Superficial Puncturing. In some instances Deep needling is close to the bone.

The strength of Deep Puncturing makes it generally inadvisable for weak patients, unless the patient has pain that is deep. When Deep Puncturing is for a weak patient, needle stimulation should be mild.

Divide *(Fen Ci)*

Divide refers to a place of division or a border. The insertion of needles in *Fen Ci* is on the border of muscles or between layers of muscles. Although points selected for *Fen Ci* all have in common the feature of location along muscle borders, the therapeutic uses of *Fen Ci* vary greatly according to the individual characteristics of points selected.

Urinary Bladder 57 *Chengshan* is located directly below the belly of the gastrocnemius muscle, in the cleft between the two heads of the gastrocnemius. As a local point, it is excellent for treating spasm of the calf muscles. Spasms may occur at night when temperatures begin to cool, during sleep when the circulation of *qi* and blood is less vigorous, or during swimming. *Chengshan* treats the acute occurrence of leg cramps, and it may be used preventatively. It also is applied for muscular pain in the low back, in the mid-back, and from the shoulders up to the occipital protuberance. Some practitioners use *Chengshan* as an Experience Point for treating spasm anywhere on the body. *Chengshan* is perhaps most famous for prevention and treatment of hemorrhoids, often combined with Urinary Bladder 60 *Kunlun*. Lastly, *Chengshan* clears and regulates the intestines and is an important point for treatment of constipation.

Urinary Bladder 58 *Feiyang* lies on the border of the gastrocnemius muscle, about one *cun* lateroinferior to *Chengshan*. *"Feiyang"* means that one's "walking is like flying," indicating that *Feiyang* is an important point to consider for walking problems. The combination of *Shenshu* Urinary Bladder 23 with *Feiyang* is useful for treating weak patients with walking problems, such as elderly patients.

Kidney 9 *Zhubin*, located at the lower end of the belly of the gastrocnemius muscle in its medial aspect, lies on a line drawn from Kidney 3 *Taixi* to Kidney 10 *Yingu*. *Zhubin* is a meeting point of the Three Leg Yin Channels, and it is the *Xi* (Cleft) Point for the Yinwei Channel. "Yinwei" means "maintenance of Yin," which also relates to lubrication and nurturing by Yin fluids, and *Zhubin* is famous for treatment of dry skin.

Large Intestine 14 *Binao* is just a little superior to the lower end of the deltoid muscle on the radial side of the humerus. A long needle inserted horizontally upward from *Binao* to Large Intestine 15 *Jianyu* lies between layers of muscles. This treats pain in the shoulder and arm, arthritis, and an inability to raise the arm at the shoulder.

Fen Ci is one of the Nine Ancient Insertion Methods based on the Nine Ancient Needles.

Short Puncturing *(Duan Ci)*

The use of Short Puncturing is associated with soreness in the bone, pain or swelling in muscle close to the bone, deep-level numbness due to Damp and Cold that is close to bony areas, and osseous rheumatism. Insertion using Short Puncturing is deep, almost to the bone.

"Short" means "gradually moving in." Although *Duan Ci* insertion is deep, the needle is inserted in short repeated intervals, rather than inserted directly to a deep level. Each time before the needle is inserted deeper, it is shaken so as to enlarge the needle hole. This promotes the elimination of pathogenic factors. Once insertion is to the desired depth, techniques of lifting, thrusting, *bu,* or *xie* may be administered. Care must be taken to never touch bone with the tip of the needle.

An interesting characteristic of *Duan Ci* is that, to the practitioner, the sensation along the acupuncture needle is simultaneously different at the tip and at the handle. This sensation is due to resistance to the needle by muscle in the affected area.

Duan Ci is one of the Twelve Ancient Methods of Insertion into the Twelve Regular Channels.

Transport *(Shu Ci)*

The word *Shu* appears frequently in acupuncture. There are the Five *Shu* Points located below the elbows and the knees, the Back-*Shu* Points along the Urinary Bladder Channel, and three different ancient acupuncture techniques called *Shu Ci*. In all instances *"Shu"* can be translated as "transport," yet in each case *Shu* has a different meaning.

This version of *Shu Ci* is one of the Twelve Ancient Methods of Insertion. Here, *"Shu"* means "disperse," which can be taken as synonymous with *xie* (Reducing). It is applied for treatment of deep pain and swelling associated with Excess, Heat, and acute conditions.

The technique is that, once there is arrival of *qi*, the needle is thrust deeply into the affected area. Once into the affected area, the needle is manipulated, then withdrawn immediately; or it is retained only a few minutes, then withdrawn. The acupuncture point is left open after the needle is withdrawn, not covered by the pressing hand. By vigorous, quick insertion and withdrawal of the needle, *Shu Ci* releases the Excess of pathogenic factors.

Few total points are chosen when using *Shu Ci* because it tends to make the patient very tired after treatment, and because taking away pathogenic factors with *xie* (Reducing) technique also causes some loss of the normal *qi*.

Bone *(Shu Gu Ci)*

Originally called *Shu Ci*, this technique is also called *Shu Gu Ci* to distinguish it from the other variations of *Shu Ci*. "*Gu*" means "bone." Of the Five Ancient Insertion Methods, this one is associated with the Kidneys, which form and dominate the bones.

Shu Gu Ci is used for treatment of problems in the bone or next to the bone: pain in the bone, Heat or Cold in bony areas, arthritis, or osseous rheumatism. Because of the close relationship of the Kidneys and the bones, treatment of these problems with *Shu Gu Ci* is improved if Reinforcing the Kidneys is part of the therapy. The needle insertion, like *Shu Ci* above for pain and swelling, is straight in and straight out. The difference is that insertion of *Shu Gu Ci* is deeper, coming very close to the bone without touching it.

In ancient times, deep needling of acupuncture points with *Shu Gu Ci* was also for treatment of the Kidneys. Kidneys are the Root of *qi* and, from a functional perspective, are the deepest (Yin) of the internal organs. Since treatment is most effective when the depth of insertion matches the level of physiological function being treated, appropriate insertion for treatment of the Kidneys is deep. Treatment related to the Lungs, such as *Ban Ci* for example, is shallow in contrast to treatment for the Kidneys with *Shu Gu Ci*.

Joint *(Guan Ci)*

Guan Ci is puncturing the portion of the tendon where the tendon ends at the joint. This is for treatment of spasm, of tendon pain, or of numbness or pain in the area of the tendon. To prevent bleeding, the acupuncture point is covered by the pressing hand as soon as the needle is withdrawn from the point. Tendons are nourished by Liver Yin and blood, and drawing blood can damage the tendon due to a loss of nourishment to the tissue. If there is pathogenic Heat in the joint, bleeding is permissible but it is not done too deeply, which can hurt the tendon.

This one of the Five Ancient Insertion Methods is associated with the Liver, which nourishes and governs the tendons. Chinese medicine views health of the tendons as synonymous with free-flowing body movement, unrestricted by pain or limited range of motion.

Relaxing *(Hui Ci)*

Hui Ci is one of the Twelve Ancient Methods of Insertion into the Twelve Regular Channels, now used for treatment of muscular ache and spasm. Originally, *Hui Ci* was for treatment of tendon *Bi*. *Bi* means there is pain resulting from obstruction in the circulation of *qi* or blood in the Channels and Collaterals due to pathogenic Wind, Cold, or Damp. One manner of classifying *Bi* is according to the locality of the distressed tissue, such as skin *Bi*, muscle *Bi*, tendon *Bi*, or bone *Bi*.

The puncturing of *Hui Ci* is near the painful muscle. The needle is shaken in the acupuncture point from front to back and from left to right in order to relax the muscle. *"Hui"* means "to enlarge," and shaking the needle enlarges the needle hole, a *xie* (Reducing) technique. "Enlarge" also has the meaning of "relaxing" the muscle and tendon. A common feature of muscular pain is spasm or contracture of muscles, which puts stress on muscle attachments, increases joint pressure, and—if protracted— can help bring about arthralgia and degenerative changes.

III. Multiple Puncturing

Multiple Puncturing employs a number of needles in order to perform a single technique, or makes use of one needle to perform multiple manipulations.

Trail *(Bao Ci)*

Trail Puncturing uses one needle to repeatedly stimulate an area which has pain that moves. The most painful point in the area is located and a needle is inserted into it. Manipulation of the needle will bring changes in the muscle, detected through the acupuncture needle as a decrease of tension in the muscle. The needle is retained in the first point until another painful trigger point is found, then the needle is withdrawn and inserted into the second point. This process is repeated by searching for and following the trail of the pain, whether it is within a diffuse area or along a meridian, and by needling into each locus of pain.

In modern times *Bao Ci* is often called Trigger Puncturing, a description which does not fully convey finding and following the trail of pain with repeated puncturing. Other names used for *Bao Ci* are Double Puncturing (Double means "add," or "to come back a second time") and Repeated Puncturing. This is one of the Twelve Ancient Methods of Insertion.

Valley *(He Gu Ci)*

Insertion using Valley Puncturing is into the indentation ("valley") between connections of muscles for treatment of muscular numbness, spasm, or pain. The needle is first inserted straight into the affected area, then drawn upward without withdrawing the needle past the surface of the skin, and inserted obliquely to the right of the original insertion. Afterward, the needle is again drawn upward without withdrawing it from the skin, and is inserted obliquely to the left of the original insertion. This manipulation may be repeated several times in a row, and may also be repeated in a series during the treatment.

He Gu Ci is also used with strong *xie* (Reducing) technique for treatment of goiter by pinching up the goiter and needling into it.

Valley Puncturing, one of the Five Ancient Insertion Methods, is associated with the Spleen, which dominates maintenance of the thickness and strength of muscles. *He Gu Ci* is not only a technique used for treatment of muscles, but is a method of needling points for treatment of the Spleen.

Even *(Ou Ci)*

"*Ou*" means "even number," or "a pair." *Ou Ci* was originally used only for treatment of angina. At first, selection of points for *Ou Ci* was based on painful points located on the upper back and chest. Significant painful points were then needled, with the same number of needles inserted in the upper chest as in the back. As the theory and practice of acupuncture developed, it was determined that the Back-*Shu* and Front-*Mu* points together is one of the most effective combinations of paired points for treatment of Heart pain, and *Ou Ci* came to mean needling of the Back-*Shu* Point and Front-*Mu* Point of the Heart for treatment of angina.

In time, *Ou Ci* was used for treatment not only of Heart pain, but for pain of any organ. Further developments of *Ou Ci* have changed it to simultaneous puncturing of the Back-*Shu* and the Front-*Mu* Point for treatment of any problem related to an organ. Other names for needling the Back-*Shu* and the Front-*Mu* Point at the same time are Yin-Yang Therapy and *Mu-Shu* Therapy. *Ou Ci* is one of the Twelve Ancient Methods of Insertion.

Team Puncturing *(Qi Ci)*

The meaning of "*Qi*" is "together," in the sense of a team effort. Three needles are used at once to amplify the force of treatment for chronic, deep, Cold pain that covers only a small area. The first needle is inserted into the center of the painful area, and the other two needles are inserted near the sides of the painful area. Since *Qi Ci*, also called Triple Puncturing (*San Ci*), is for treatment of chronic Cold *Bi*, it is often used with moxa. Also, needles are retained for a longer time due to the presence of Cold. The effects of multiple deep needling can be very strong for the patient, so *Qi Ci* is not often used. *Qi Ci* is one of the Twelve Ancient Methods of Insertion into the Twelve Regular Channels.

Light *(Yang Ci)*

Yang Ci is sometimes called Amplified Puncturing because it uses five needles at once. *"Yang"* means "superficial," "light." Light Puncturing is for treatment of acute *Bi* pain from stagnated Cold that is superficial and covers a large area. The insertion is only a little deeper than Superficial Puncturing and needle stimulation is "light"—from mild to none. One needle is inserted into the center of the affected area and then the other four needles are placed around it at the corners of the painful area.

Yang Ci is one of the Twelve Ancient Methods of Insertion.

Strengthen *(Bang Ci)*

Bang Ci is insertion of a needle into a point, followed by oblique insertion of a second needle nearby in one of two ways. The second needle is either angled toward the first so that the tips of the two needles meet, or it is inserted near the first needle and angled obliquely away from it. *"Bang"* literally means "near." *Bang Ci* is used as a means of strengthening the therapeutic effects of an acupuncture point with the addition of a second needle. *Bang* is sometimes also translated as "Added" or "Double," meaning "added effect," or "double the effect."

Bang Ci is for treatment of chronic localized pain that is not severe. Patients with such symptoms often are Deficient and exhibit low body function, so one needle is added to strengthen the effects of treatment. Two examples of this type of treatment are Large Intestine 15 *Jianyu* combined with Sanjiao 14 *Jianliao* for shoulder pain or for an inability to move the shoulder joint, and *Xiyan* (Extra Points), a pair of points to the sides of the patellar ligament, for pain or coldness of the knee.

Bang Ci is one of the Twelve Ancient Methods of Insertion into the Twelve Regular Channels.

IV. Bleeding

Bleeding of acupuncture points is for removing pathogenic Heat or pathogenic *qi*. Extra caution is advised when bleeding Deficient patients.

Collateral Puncturing *(Luo Ci)*

Luo Ci is surface puncturing with a three-edged needle. Some modern practitioners use a large gauge filiform needle instead of a three-edged needle. Insertion is just under the skin surface and into veins to cause bleeding. The needle is withdrawn immediately after insertion and the point is squeezed to draw a small amount of blood. *Luo Ci* is for treatment of conditions such as high fever, mania, sore throat, localized congestion or swelling, high blood pressure, severe headache, or red and painful eyes. This is one of the Nine Ancient Insertion Methods based on the Nine Ancient Needles.

Bleeding *Taiyang* (Extra Point) is for Excess type stroke and for high blood pressure. Urinary Bladder 40 *Weizhong* is famous for bleeding to treat severe back pain. Bleeding *Weizhong* is also for toxic Heat in the blood, such as blood poisoning or conditions with simultaneous vomiting and diarrhea. Bleeding the *Jing*-Well points or the *Shixuan* (Extra Points) treats Excess type stroke. Lung 5 *Chize* is bled for hemoptysis, and bleeding Pericardium 3 *Quze* treats chest pain due to blood congestion. Bleeding the ear apex is an Experience Point for treatment of red, painful eyes, and of children's high fever.

Sometimes, cupping is combined with *Luo Ci* to promote drawing blood from the point.

Assistant *(Zan Ci)*

Originally, *Zan Ci* was for treatment of abscesses and carbuncles by puncturing the affected area shallowly and repeatedly with a three-edged needle to cause bleeding. *Zan Ci* is sometimes called Repeated Shallow Puncturing. *"Zan"* means "to support" or "to assist," and its purpose is to assist the removal of superficial pathogenic Heat. Modern use of *Zan Ci* is for treatment of skin problems with pathogenic Heat, such as herpes zoster.

This is one of the Twelve Ancient Methods of Insertion.

Leopard *(Bao Wen Ci)*

The original use of *Bao Wen Ci* was to bleed small vessels and evacuate stagnated blood to treat Heart disease or illness due to obstruction in the meridians. It is currently used for skin problems with pathogenic Heat with symptoms such as red spots, itching, or multiple abscesses. It is similar to *Zan Ci* except that it is for treatment of problems that cover a larger area.

Leopard Puncturing is so named because of the heavy spotting of the skin that results from this bleeding technique. *Bao Wen Ci* is one of the Five Ancient Needling Methods, associated with the Heart, which dominates the blood.

Heavy Reducing *(Da Xie Ci)*

Very few, if any, acupuncturists in the West have training in Heavy Puncturing. It is one of the Nine Ancient Needling Methods, used to drain pus and blood from large abscesses, boils, and carbuncles. The ancient needle used for *Da Xie Ci* was sword-shaped, while the modern needle resembles a surgical chisel.

V. Follow the Channel Puncturing

Points are selected according to diagnosis of meridian and organ symptomatology.

Channel Puncturing (Jing Ci)

Points are chosen to eliminate blockage on a given channel or its proximal area by treating stasis or obstruction of *qi* or blood. Commonly, *xie* (Reducing) technique is applied for conditions of obstruction. *Jing Ci* also is the needling of points corresponding to the channel of an organ affected by disease.

A prescription for nasal congestion and difficulty breathing is *Yingxiang* Large Intestine 20 combined with *Hegu* Large Intestine 4. A prescription for nasal congestion or sinus inflammation is Gall Bladder 15 Head-*Linqi* plus *Yintang* (Extra Point).

An example of *Jing Ci* for treatment according to the organ and to the channel pathway is Liver 3 *Taichong* for vertex headache and for headaches that affect the eyes.

Channel Puncturing is one of the Nine Ancient Needling Methods based on uses of the Nine Ancient Needles.

Transport (Shu Point Puncturing, Shu Ci)

Two varieties of *Shu Ci* previously mentioned were both in the Deep Puncturing category. This version of *Shu Ci* is needling of acupuncture points which convey their effects directly to their related organs. Points originally selected for *Shu Ci* were the Five *Shu* Points on the extremities distal to the elbows and knees, and the Back-*Shu* Points on the Urinary

Bladder meridian. Acupuncture points later included in *Shu Ci* are the Inferior *He*-Sea Points, the *Yuan* (Source) Points, and the *Xi* (Cleft) Points because insertion into these points has a direct effect on their related organs. This is one of the Nine Ancient Insertion Methods.

Yin Puncturing *(Yin Ci)*

The first use of *Yin Ci* was for Cold type syncope, with symptoms of extreme bodily cold, cold and numb extremities, pale or gray facial color, lingering abdominal pain that prevents the patient from lying straight, and a pulse that is deep, slow, and so weak it can hardly be palpated. Symptoms of collapse, a breakdown in strength or health thereby causing a cessation of normal body functions, are associated with collapse of Yin according to Chinese medicine since it is the nutritive aspect of Yin that supports the Yang aspect of body functions.

The Kidney is the source of the Yin and Yang of the whole body, and Yin Puncturing uses only one acupuncture point, bilateral insertion at Kidney 3 *Taixi*. Due to the patient's extreme weakness, only very mild stimulation is used, just inducing the arrival of *qi (de qi)*. What is most unusual about *Yin Ci* is the length of treatment: needles are retained from one half hour up to three hours. *Taixi* is the only acupuncture point that Reinforces patients when needles are retained for such a long time.

Yin Ci is now used to treat any kind of weakness and is combined with other points to treat a wider range of conditions. For unchecked sweating, *Taixi* is combined with *Hegu* Large Intestine 4. Stomach 36 *Zusanli* and *Taixi* are used together for treatment of weak patients with high blood pressure. The Kidney is closely related to the Heart, and *Taixi* may be combined with *Neiguan* Pericardium 6 for Heart problems. Insomnia indicates a problem with the Heart, and one prescription for insomnia is *Taixi, Neiguan,* and *Shenmen* Heart 7. Any time a treatment requires that needles be retained for a long time, it is possible to add *Yin Ci* to the prescription.

Yin Ci is one of the Twelve Ancient Methods of Needling into the Twelve Regular Channels.

VI. Diverse Puncturing

Diverse Puncturing makes use of acupuncture points distant from the location of a disease. Selection of points can sometimes seem unusual due to their differences in location from the disease condition.

Remote Puncturing *(Yuan Dao Ci)*
"Yuan" means "far." Remote Puncturing selects points far from the location where disease occurs. For problems in the lower body, points in the upper body may be selected and vice versa. Acupuncture points distal to the elbows and knees are generally considered the most effective points for treating problems located on the torso or head.

Some examples are: Du 20 *Baihui* for any kind of prolapse, or for gastrointestinal pain; Liver 1 *Dadun* for hernia, orchitis, or menorrhagia; Lung 5 *Chize* for cough or asthma; Kidney 1 *Yongquan* for vertex headache or coma; Small Intestine 3 *Houxi* for hypochondriac pain or sciatic pain; Du 16 *Fengfu* for pain or motor difficulties in the lower extremities. Large Intestine 4 *Hegu* is considered the master point for the head and face and is one of the most important points to include in prescriptions for conditions such as headache, sinus problems, facial paralysis, toothache, or dizziness.

Remote Puncturing is one of the Nine Ancient Insertion Methods based on uses of the Nine Ancient Needles.

Giant Puncturing *(Ju Ci)*

Giant Puncturing is mainly indicated when a problem occurs on one side of the body and the abnormal pulse is on the opposite side. When there is disease, the abnormal pulse ordinarily is on the same side as the problem. This change in the position of the pulse indicates that the problem is moving to the opposite side. If there is a problem on the right but the affected pulse is on the left, then needle insertion is on the left side.

Acupuncture technique for *Ju Ci* is with *bu* and *xie* according to Excess and Deficient symptoms. If, for example, there is weakness on the right side, the left side may be treated with *xie* (Reducing) technique to balance the two sides of the body. The use of Giant Puncturing to balance the two sides of the body has developed to include selection of points on the side opposite the location of the condition even when the disease condition and the abnormal pulse are on the same side, such as in the case of stroke patients. *Ju Ci* strictly selects points from the *jing mai* (the Twelve Regular Channels and the Eight Extra Channels), and does not make use of *Ahshi* Points.

This is one of the Nine Ancient Insertion Methods.

Peculiar Puncturing *(Miu Ci)*

Miu Ci is selected when there are acute symptoms but the pulse has not yet manifested any abnormalities. This indicates the problem is still superficial and light, not serious. In contrast to Giant Puncturing, which is insertion into points in the *jing mai*, Peculiar Puncturing is insertion into *Luo* (Connecting) Points or along the Connecting Channel (*luo mai*). Peculiar Puncturing also makes use of local points (*Ahshi* Points). Like Giant Puncturing, *Miu Ci* inserts needles on the side opposite the problem.

Peculiar Puncturing was so named because the location of needles seemed strange from the patient's point of view. It would seem most peculiar, for example, to treat a swollen and painful acutely sprained ankle by administering treatment on the healthy ankle—which is exactly what is done with *Miu Ci.*

Modern uses of *Miu Ci* include contralateral puncturing of *Jing*-Well Points as well as bleeding small superficial veins for treatment of blood stasis.

Other Techniques

Through and Through Puncturing *(Tou Ci)*

The special feature of *Tou Ci* is the use of few insertion points, and the needle passes through two or more acupuncture points or meridians. The tip of the needle should never emerge from the skin when using Through and Through Puncturing, for not only are the therapeutic effects of needling not obtained, but normal *qi* is lost in the process. The stimulation of Through and Through insertion is strong, and the sensation is profound. *Tou Ci* is closely associated with two of the Nine Ancient Needles, the Long Needle and the Large Needle, and dates back to Neolithic times when more effects had to be obtained from fewer needles. Modern use of *Tou Ci* is often for treatment of paralysis and numbness.

To obtain greater therapeutic effect from a single needle, insertion at *Neiguan* Pericardium 6 can be all the way to the other side of the forearm, in the area of *Waiguan* Sanjiao 5. *Neiguan* is a very powerful point and its needling sensation can be too strong for some patients. In such cases it is possible to obtain the same therapeutic effects without such strong needle sensation by inserting from the other direction, from *Waiguan* to *Neiguan*.

Heart 7 *Shenmen* is an important point for any Heart problem, and its effects can be amplified by inserting from *Shenmen* to Pericardium 7 *Daling*. This version of Through and Through Puncturing is accomplished by inserting under the ulnar side of the tendon of m. flexor carpi ulnaris.

Conditions of Liver Excess can be treated by using Kidney 1 *Yongquan*. However, *Yongquan* is one of the most sensitive points of all, so instead, insertion can be Through and Through from Liver 3 *Taichong* to *Yongquan*.

Treatment to fortify both Kidney Yin and Kidney Yang at the same time can be obtained by needling horizontally from Urinary Bladder 23 *Shenshu* to Du 4 *Mingmen*.

Insertion at Urinary Bladder 1 *Jingming*, a sensitive point, can be frightening to patients because of its nearness to the eye. An effective alternative to perpendicular insertion into *Jingming* is Through and Through Puncturing from Urinary Bladder 2 *Zanzhu* to *Jingming*.

Flame Needle Puncturing *(Cui Ci)*

It is most unlikely any practitioners outside of China practice Flame Needle Puncturing, called "Tempered Puncturing" in the *Nei Jing*. *Cui Ci*, one of the Nine Ancient Insertion Methods based on uses of the Nine Ancient Needles, originally was used for treating numbness and Cold of the bones.

According to the *Nei Jing*: "First burn the needle to red, then insert for treatment of Cold or numbness."

The needle used for *Cui Ci* is long, from three to four *cun* in length, and thicker than an ordinary needle, from one half millimeter to one millimeter in diameter. In ancient times the needle was made from copper, selected for its ability to conduct heat. The needle was heated over a burning coal until it was glowing hot, then inserted quickly to the desired depth and withdrawn immediately. The handle of the original needle was made from bamboo or from bone to protect the practitioner's fingers from burning. In modern times, Flame Needling is mainly used for treatment of lymphadenitis, carbuncles, elephantiasis, and abscesses. Insertion of *Cui Ci* should not be too deep. It is inadvisable for use in areas with a lot of blood vessels, and is not done on the torso, just the extremities.

There is also a Cutaneous Flame Needle for tapping on the skin. The number of needles in the head of the hammer can vary from three to nine. The needle tips of the hammer are finer than that of the Flame Needle used for deep needling, but are thicker than that of an ordinary Cutaneous Needle. Tapping with a Cutaneous Flame Needle is often used for rheumatic pain, for pain in the joints that is not deep, and for some stubborn skin problems such as scabies or psoriasis. Tapping may also be used for cold or numbness of skin or muscle; if the affected area is not too large, a single, short Flame Needle can be inserted and quickly withdrawn. When tapping the skin with a Cutaneous Flame Needle, the hammering cannot be too light, which would have no effect, or too heavy, which would cause burning.

Combined Needling Techniques

Frequently, needling techniques are combined to meet a patient's needs rather than applied singly.

Insertion at Stomach 38 *Tiaokou* is Remote Puncturing for shoulder pain and inability to raise the arm at the shoulder. Insertion to the normal depth at *Tiaokou*, up to one *cun*, may not be effective enough, and treatment can be enhanced by combining Remote Puncturing with Through and Through Puncturing by needling deeply from *Tiaokou* to *Chengshan* Urinary Bladder 57.

Heel pain is treated with Pericardium 7 *Daling* by inserting on the side opposite the pain. This is a combination of Remote Puncturing with Giant Puncturing.

Jing Ci (Channel Puncturing to remove blockage along a channel pathway and its surrounding area) by itself likely does not have a heavy enough effect for treatment of migraine headaches. Insertion of a needle from *Taiyang* (Extra Point) to *Shuaigu* Gall Bladder 8 combines *Jing Ci* with Through and Through Puncturing. The addition of a needle into Gall Bladder 41 Foot-*Linqi* provides the further effects of Remote Puncturing. In this way, three types of needle insertion are achieved with the use of two acupuncture points.

One final example of combining techniques is the treatment of a thirty-five-year-old patient who had rheumatic fever at age thirteen, and had suffered general fatigue ever since. He came for treatment of left hand and forearm pain, which had become so strong and so constant that he was waking a number of times during the night. The patient's complexion was pale and sallow, his voice was soft, and his pulses were slow, deep, and weak. Due to the patient's obvious weakness, the treatment plan was to use only one needle if possible. A fine gauge needle was inserted in the affected arm from *Waiguan* Sanjiao 5 Through and Through to *Neiguan* Pericardium 6, with the patient feeling only a slight effect from the presence of the needle. Since the response to needling was light, *Tou Ci* was combined with *Bang Ci* when a second needle was inserted near the first and angled away from it so that the tip of the second needle went to Pericardium 5 *Jianshi*. The patient then experienced *qi* sensation into the hand as well as up the forearm and to the chest. When he returned for treatment the next day the patient had experienced a reduction in the pain, and he had undisturbed sleep the night after the first treatment.

Different types of needle insertions combined with the various ways of manipulating needles—such as *bu*, *xie*, and Even techniques—can cover a wide range of clinical uses. Permutations derived from different configurations of these various methods are limited only by a practitioner's insights and inventiveness.

Chart 7-4a.

SIX TYPES OF INSERTION
ACCORDING TO THE *NEI JING*

I. **Shallow** **Puncturing**	Hair Puncturing *Mao Ci*	9 Needles
	Half Puncturing *Ban Ci*	5 *Zang*
	Floating Puncturing *Fu Ci*	12 Methods
	Straight In Puncturing *Zhi Ci*	12 Methods
II. **Deep** **Puncturing**	Divide Puncturing *Fen Ci*	9 Needles
	Short Puncturing *Duan Ci*	12 Methods
	Transport Puncturing *Shu Ci*	12 Methods
	Bone Puncturing *Shu Gu Ci*	5 *Zang*
	Joint Puncturing *Guan Ci*	5 *Zang*
	Relaxing Puncturing *Hui Ci*	12 Methods
III. **Multiple** **Puncturing**	Trail Puncturing *Bao Ci*	12 Methods
	Valley Puncturing *He Gu Ci*	5 *Zang*
	Even Puncturing *Ou Ci*	12 Methods
	Team Puncturing *Qi Ci*	12 Methods
	Light Puncturing *Yang Ci*	12 Methods
	Strengthen Puncturing *Bang Ci*	12 Methods
IV. **Bleeding**	Collateral Puncturing *Luo Ci*	9 Needles
	Assistant Puncturing *Zan Ci*	12 Methods
	Leopard Puncturing *Bao Wen Ci*	5 *Zang*
	Heavy Puncturing *Da Xie Ci*	9 Needles
V. **Follow the** **Channel**	Channel Puncturing *Jing Ci*	9 Needles
	Shu Point Puncturing *Shu Ci*	9 Needles
	Yin Puncturing *Yin Ci*	12 Methods
VI. **Diverse** **Puncturing**	Remote Puncturing *Yuan Dao Ci*	9 Needles
	Giant Puncturing *Ju Ci*	9 Needles
	Peculiar Puncturing *Miu Ci*	*

Chart 7-4b.

OTHER TECHNIQUES

Through and Through Puncturing *Tou Ci*	*
Flame Needle Puncturing *Cui Ci*	9 Needles

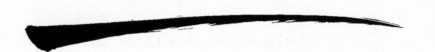

8.

Bu, Xie, and Even Technique

Bu and Xie

Once points have been selected to form a prescription, treatment is administered with the Proper Technique. There are so many possible techniques to select that making a choice can seem complex. In addition to needling methods based on the Nine Ancient Needles, the twelve different techniques for needling into the Twelve Regular Channels, and needling methods associated with each of the *zang* organs, there are other techniques that have not been mentioned. Furthermore, most of these ancient needling methods can be applied with either *bu* (Reinforcing) or *xie* (Reducing) techniques, or some combination of *bu* and *xie* together. As a consequence, questions arise whether to use only *bu* or only *xie*, whether to use *xie* before *bu* or to use *bu* before *xie*, and when to use Even technique *(ping bu ping xie)*.

Since there are so many factors to keep in mind, it helps to keep everything as simple as possible. The *Nei Jing* advises that diagnosis designates the Proper Technique. In theory the main cause of disease is the imbalance of Yin and Yang, and the general plan of treatment is to balance the whole body, not just treat the symptoms. When there is *shi* (Excess) the pathogen is strong and when there is *xu* (Deficiency) the patient's *qi* is less than normal. Chronic conditions mean there is lowered resistance, while acute conditions result from the influence of pathogenic factors. Moreover, pathogenic factors can be either *shi* or *xu;* and pathogenic factors may be external or internal. An example of *shi* pathogens is pain and swelling at the same time. Two examples of *xu* pathogens are numbness, and whole body itching without an apparent cause. Internal pathogenic factors result from mental or emotional influences, such as a sudden emotional shock for example. Pathogenic factors of whatever origin can cause any of a myriad physical responses based on a patient's constitutional predisposition to disease. This is in accordance with the *Nei Jing* theory, "Where there is Deficiency is where pathogens may reside."

In conditions of *xu* (Deficiency) the treatment plan is to Reinforce the patient's *qi;* for *shi* (Excess) conditions, the plan is to Reduce the excess of pathogenic factors. In the *Nei Jing* this is concisely expressed, "For Deficiency, add; for Excess, take away." The classical Chinese word for "add" (*"ji,"* "to save," "to restore") is synonymous with *bu* (Reinforcing); and *"duo"* ("to take away," "to seize") is synonymous with *xie* (Reducing). These classical terms *"ji"* and *"duo"* are not part of modern medical parlance and have been completely replaced by the use of *bu* and *xie*.

According to the *Nei Jing*, it is axiomatic that of all the possible acupuncture techniques that can be used for treatment, the two most important are *bu* and *xie*. The purpose of *bu* is to fortify the patient so that the *qi* is ample. This causes a pushing up and out of *qi*, analogous to filling a vessel to overflowing. The result of *bu* is to correct deficiency of vital function and to strengthen the body's resistance. Use of *xie* is to Reduce pathogens and to eliminate the Excess of pathogenic factors.

There are three important details to keep in mind when applying *bu* or *xie* techniques. First is the relative strength of the stimulation. Second is time, or the length of the treatment. Third is the method, or specific type of technique employed. Of these three, the most important is the strength of the treatment. *Bu* is mild treatment with the needles retained for a suitable time, generally no longer than fifteen minutes. This method is for the patient who exhibits weakness. *Xie* is generally associated with strong treatment regardless of whether the amount of time the needles are retained is long or short. *Xie* is indicated for acute problems, for Excess, and for pain. Pain means there is blockage or obstruction and requires a relatively stronger treatment, in some cases even bleeding of acupuncture points, in order to restore normal circulation.

It can be said that the general purpose of acupuncture techniques is to help balance the Yin and Yang functions of the body, and to promote normal circulation of *qi* and blood in the Channels and Collaterals. Keep in mind, however, that for any technique to have its effect there must first be arrival of *qi (de qi)*. Another important consideration is risk to the patient. Famous physicians, such as the great Hua Tuo, have set examples of acupuncture practiced cautiously yet with excellent results.

Twelve Methods of *Bu* and *Xie*

A summary of *bu* and *xie* techniques in the *Ling Shu* lists four pairs of *bu* and *xie* methods as the most important. They are based on: 1) breathing; 2) the speed with which needles are inserted and withdrawn; 3) "opening" and "closing" of the acupuncture points when needles are taken out; and 4) strength of treatment. Since these four methods are listed as foremost in the *Ling Shu*, they will be discussed first.

Strong and Mild

Even though views and schools of thought differ as to what constitutes *bu* or *xie*, most agree that strong stimulation of an acupuncture point is a *xie* (Reducing) technique, and mild stimulation is a *bu* (Reinforcing) technique. According to the *Ling Shu*, "When pulse diagnosis shows the meridian *qi* is Deficient, follow and restore *(ji)*." The word "follow" means "to adhere to" the diagnosis of Deficiency, implying use of mild treatment. As we have already seen, "restore" *("ji")* is synonymous with *bu*.

Conversely, according to the *Ling Shu*, "When pulse diagnosis shows the meridian *qi* is Excessive, face it and take away *(duo)*." "Face" the Excess means "to overcome by confronting" it with active means. English has the same meaning when we say someone "faces" a problem. Overcoming the Excess is accomplished by strong technique since *"duo"* means more than "take away," it explicitly means "take by force."

Cover and Uncover (Closed and Open)

In the second most used method of *bu* and *xie*, at the time that needles are taken out, acupuncture points are either pressed with the pressing hand (Cover) or not pressed (Uncover). Uncover, also called "leaving the point open," is a Reducing technique because it allows pathogenic *qi* to escape when the needle is taken out. According to the *Nei Jing*, in Uncover technique the needle is shaken as it is being withdrawn. This allows more pathogenic *qi* to come out with the needle. Pressing on the acupuncture point with the pressing hand as soon as the needle is taken out (Cover) is a Reinforcing technique since it helps to retain the Vital *qi*.

Quick and Slow

The basis of Quick and Slow is that *qi* easily moves in the same direction as the needle when the needle is moved slowly. When the needle is moved quickly, it is difficult for *qi* to move with the needle and to keep up with it.

The purpose of *xie* (Reducing) is to draw pathogenic *qi* up and out to disperse it. Reducing with Quick and Slow means, after arrival of *qi* (*de qi*), quick insertion to the desired depth and slow withdrawal of the needle. Quick and Slow can be applied to the initial insertion and final withdrawal of needles, and also to techniques of repeated lifting and thrusting while needles are retained during treatment.

An ancient meaning of *bu* is "add," and the purpose of Reinforcing is to fill the *qi* and restore it to a healthy level. Quick and Slow as a *bu* technique means slow insertion and quick withdrawal of needles, or slow thrusting and quick lifting of needles when repeatedly lifting and thrusting. The slow insertion helps to add to the *qi,* in the way that pouring liquid into a container fills it. Drawing the needle upward quickly and lightly prevents Vital *qi* from coming out.

Breathing

The principle of Breathing as a *bu* or *xie* technique is based on the relationship of breath to the flow of *qi* in meridians. We already saw in Chapter 2 that each complete inhalation and exhalation moves *qi* and blood in the meridians six *cun* (six Chinese proportional inches). In addition, inhaling and exhaling have distinctly different effects on *qi* in the meridians, and we can take advantage of this for the purpose of *bu* and *xie*.

Reducing is accomplished by inserting the needle and obtaining the arrival of *qi* while the patient begins to inhale. If *qi* does not arrive when the needle is first inserted, the practitioner needs to wait until the next breath and obtain the arrival of *qi* with the inhalation. Inhaling holds *qi* in place inside the meridians, which enables pathogenic *qi* to be grasped by the *qi* around the needle. When pathogenic *qi* is captured in this way, it can be Reduced. The needle is withdrawn with the beginning of exhalation and must be completely taken out by the end of exhalation. Exhaling helps the elimination of pathogenic *qi*.

Reinforcing is accomplished by inserting the needle and obtaining the arrival of *qi* while the patient exhales, and taking the needle out with the inhalation. Exhaling helps the elimination of waste *qi* and allows more of the normal *qi* to enter the meridians. In this way, inserting the needle during exhalation helps the normal *qi* to enter the meridians and to flourish. Since inhaling holds *qi* in place inside the meridians, withdrawing the needle while inhaling serves to retain the Vital *qi* and prevent it from escaping as the needle is taken out.

Lift and Thrust

Lifting and Thrusting of needles for *bu* and *xie* is a combination of two methods already mentioned: Strong and Mild, and Quick and Slow.

Bu is lightly and quickly lifting needles and thrusting slowly. There is more stimulus during the thrusting of the needle than during lifting, but the stimulus is still mild.

Xie is thrusting quickly and lifting slowly. The stimulus of Lifting and Thrusting for *xie* is strong.

Three Levels

Acupuncture points have three levels of depth: upper (*"Tian,"* "heaven"), middle (*"Ren,"* "man"), and deep (*"Di,"* "earth"). The different manners of lifting and thrusting needles through the three levels, with differences in stimulation at the three levels, can result in either a *bu* or a *xie* technique.

Three Levels Down is called in Chinese *Shao Shan Huo*, "Set the whole mountain on fire." Now used as a *bu* technique for many different problems, it was originally used to lift the Yang for treatment of Cold symptoms. After insertion and arrival of *qi*, the needle is inserted to the first level *(Tian)*. While pausing briefly at the first level, the needle is rotated back and forth to mildly stimulate the acupuncture point. The needle is then inserted to the middle level *(Ren)* and stimulated briefly, and finally inserted to the deep level *(Di)* and stimulated. The needle is inserted gradually inward, level by level, then lifted up to the first level in one light, quick movement. Once at the first level, the whole sequence may be repeated as much as the practitioner considers appropriate.

Three Levels Up for *xie* is called *Tou Tian Liang*, "All the sky cooling." Originally, *Tou Tian Liang* was used for treatment of conditions with Heat, including problems such as high fever. As soon as there is arrival of *qi*, the needle is inserted to the deep level. The needle is then lifted gradually level by level, with brief stimulation of the acupuncture point at each of the three levels. The sequence may be repeated, with quick insertion to the deep level and slow lifting of the needle level by level. To emphasize the *xie* nature of *Tou Tian Liang*, stimulus of the technique can be strong.

Originally, Three Levels Up and Three Levels Down were used for treatment of Heat and Cold cases respectively. High level of skill at performing the Three Levels has since come to be considered the pinnacle of *bu* and *xie* technique for treatment of any condition.

Follow and Against

To the following quote from the *Nei Jing* some practitioners have given a different interpretation than what we have seen above for Strong and Mild: "When pulse diagnosis shows the meridian *qi* is Deficient, follow and restore. When pulse diagnosis shows the meridian *qi* is Excessive, face it and take it away." This has been taken to mean that *bu* is insertion of needles in the direction in which the *qi* of the channel flows, and that *xie* is insertion against the flow of the channel. Though it has already been shown with the techniques of Strong and Mild that this is not the original meaning of this passage in the *Nei Jing*, there is merit to Follow and Against as techniques for *bu* and *xie*.

We can see that the angle of insertion in relation to the meridian does have an effect on *qi* when we consider some advice by Yang Ji-Zhou.

His recommendation is that needles not be inserted perfectly perpendicular into the channels because this damages the *qi* by impeding *qi* flow.

Although there is value to Follow and Against for *bu* and *xie*, the other methods already mentioned are of greater importance. And, Follow and Against has its limitations. For example, needle insertion into meridians on the chest and upper back can only be horizontally or obliquely downward for safety reasons, regardless of the direction in which the *qi* flows in those channels. Moreover, the effects of other methods of *bu* and *xie* can predominate in spite of the direction of insertion in relation to the flow of *qi* in the meridians. This means that insertion of a needle from *Dazhui* Du 14 to *Taodao* Du 13 (against the flow of the channel), combined with the technique of *Shao Shan Huo* ("Setting the Whole Mountain on Fire," or Three Levels Down), will have a Reinforcing effect.

An entirely different use of the direction of needle insertion is derived from a *Nei Jing* technique called *Dao Qi*. Needles are aimed in the direction of the problem that is being treated—pointed up to treat the upper body and down to treat the lower body, without any regard for the direction of the *qi* flow in the meridians. The angle of insertion is used only to direct treatment to the upper or lower body and in itself has no *bu* or *xie* effect. An example of this is needle insertion at Lung 7 *Lieque*. For treatment of the Lung, needles inserted into *Lieque* are directed up the arm toward the body. When *Lieque* is used for treatment of the thumb, needles are inserted down toward the hand.

Duration

Bu and *xie* are very flexible when determined by the amount of time that needles are retained. It can be generally said that *bu* is retaining needles for a short time, up to twenty minutes maximum; longer than twenty minutes is *xie*. However, when the strength of needle stimulation is strong, the effect is *xie*, even if the needles are retained for only a short time. Also, when the strength of treatment is strong, it is generally advisable that needles not be retained too long. One exception is treatment of muscle spasm. Treatment in this case is needles retained for a long time combined with strong stimulation.

Another exception is treatment of neurasthenia. Strength of treatment for neurasthenia is very light and needles are retained for about half an hour. The reason the needles are retained for such a long time is that prolonged light stimulus of acupuncture points which affect the nervous system, such as Heart 7 *Shenmen*, helps restore the normal polarization of nerve fibers. In healthy conditions the stimulus of a single nerve impulse is enough to repolarize nerve fibers. In the case of neurasthenia, nerves cannot quickly recover ionic balance, so light stimulus for an extended time is needed to repolarize nerves and return them to a resting state.

Number of Needles

The burden that treatment places on the patient's overall *qi* is proportional to the number of needles inserted during a treatment. Fewer needles is *bu*; more needles is *xie*.

Rotation

After the arrival of *qi*, needles can be retained and stimulated by rotating them in place. Mild strength of rotation is *bu*; strong stimulus of rotation is *xie*.

Turning

Turning needles in a clockwise or a counterclockwise direction to produce a *bu* or a *xie* effect is a technique that was used more in the past and is seldom used in modern times. There are differences in treatment for men and women, and also for the time of day. It is possible that keeping all this in mind can make Turning seem too complicated. Few practitioners use Turning as a primary method of *bu* and *xie*.

The direction of Turning for *bu* and *xie* changes according to the time of day, because men have more *qi* in the upper body in the morning hours and more *qi* in the lower body in the afternoon.

The complete opposite is true for women, who have more *qi* in the lower body in the morning and more *qi* in the upper body in the afternoon. This leads to methods of Turning for women that are opposite to those for men.

The following charts list the different methods of Turning:

Chart 8-1a.

TURNING AS A *BU* TECHNIQUE FOR MEN

morning	clockwise
afternoon	counterclockwise

Chart 8-1b.

TURNING AS A *XIE* TECHNIQUE FOR MEN

morning	counterclockwise
afternoon	clockwise

Chart 8-2a.

TURNING AS A *BU* TECHNIQUE FOR WOMEN

morning	counterclockwise
afternoon	clockwise

Chart 8-2b.

TURNING AS A *XIE* TECHNIQUE FOR WOMEN

morning	clockwise
afternoon	counterclockwise

In addition, it can be difficult to reconcile methods of Turning for *bu* or *xie* when combined with a different method of turning needles which is used to direct treatment to different parts of the body. In the latter case, turning needles clockwise is used to direct *qi* to the upper body, while turning the needle counterclockwise directs *qi* to the lower body.

There is more to these different techniques than merely turning the needles in one direction or another. Important factors such as the speed and strength of turning can control the effects of these techniques. One style of applying Turning for *bu* or *xie* is large turns of the needle in the desired direction, done with light stimulation. In contrast, a style of Turning for directing the *qi* up or down employs slow, small turns of the needle while the needle is grasped with force by the needling hand.

Because these different methods of turning needles—for *bu* or *xie*, and for directing *qi* up or down—can create contradictions or confusion in the minds of practitioners, they are seldom used.

Midnight-Noon Law

The Midnight-Noon Law (*Zi Wu Liu Zhu*, "Midnight-noon ebb and flow") for *bu* and *xie* is mentioned for reference only. This is an ancient method of selecting acupuncture points based on the flow and ebb of *qi* and blood along different meridians. These changes are believed to be related to designated days and hours in terms of Heavenly Stems and Earthly Branches of the lunar calendar. Prediction of the ebb or flow of acupuncture points is used to select which points can be used for treatment to *xie* ("ebb," "to take away") or *bu* ("flow," "to add").

Even Technique

Even technique in Chinese is expressed as *"ping bu ping xie."* *"Ping"* means "equal amount" or "even." Even technique means that both *bu* and *xie* are applied to an acupuncture point during a treatment. It is frequently used for patients with a mixture of Excess and Deficient conditions, and for treating pain. There are different schools of thought and opinions on application of Even technique.

Even Technique According to Chen Hui

Prior to Yang Ji-Zhou, the prevailing style of Even treatment had been to first apply *xie* technique, then follow with *bu*. Although this had been the style of Even technique for many centuries, Chen Hui was the first to provide a theoretical explanation.

According to Chen Hui, it is necessary to first apply *xie* in order to eliminate pathogenic factors. To *bu* first would Reinforce pathogenic factors rather than Reduce them. Moreover, first Reducing pathogenic factors provides more room for normal *qi* to enter. *Xie* to Reduce pathogenic factors first also applies to elimination of waste *qi*. *Qi* is a fundamental substance and, like any other aspect of the body's metabolism, it develops waste products that need to be eliminated. Opening a treatment with *xie* to first eliminate waste *qi* enables more of the normal *qi* to enter the meridians when they are filled by *bu* technique.

Although most practitioners now follow the developments made by Yang Ji-Zhou, there are still practitioners influenced by the thinking of Chen Hui.

Even Technique According to Yang Ji-Zhou

When applying Even technique, Yang Ji-Zhou adhered to an ancient meaning of the word *"ping,"* which translates as "light" or "mild." This very mild application of Even technique as developed by Yang Ji-Zhou was an innovation in treatment for weak and delicate patients because, even though it uses both *bu* and *xie,* the stimulation of the technique is very mild.

Another development of Even technique by Yang Ji-Zhou is that not only are *bu* and *xie* mild, they can both be administered during the same manipulation of the needle ("evenly") rather than at separate times. A simple variation of this is lifting and thrusting of needles with even strength of manipulation in both up and down directions. Another variation of this approach to Even technique is rotation of a needle back and forth with even stimulation in both directions and equal-sized turns in each direction.

Developments of Yang Ji-Zhou's use of mild *bu* and mild *xie* to administer Even technique created the possibility of mild Reducing treatment. Prior to Yang Ji-Zhou, *xie* (Reducing) was generally associated with strong treatment. Due to the insights of Yang Ji-Zhou, any of the various *xie* techniques can be administered within a wider range of stimulation—from very strong to very light. Mild *xie* is accomplished by relying on the style of needle manipulation (e.g., Three Levels Up) rather than the strength of manipulation to deliver *xie* technique. Due to Yang Ji-Zhou, innovations in Even technique ultimately provided greater nuance and subtlety of both *bu* and *xie* treatment.

Some Uses of Even Technique

Mild Even technique can be a very useful approach to the treatment of pain. After the arrival of *qi*, needles may be rotated lightly back and forth until the patient has some sensation of *qi* moving along the meridian. In successive manipulations of needles as the treatment goes on, the strength of rotation gradually increases, though needle sensation remains light to the patient, who develops insensitivity to this procedure. Pain indicates blockage or obstruction. Light Even treatment such as this has been found effective for the treatment of pain because it promotes the circulation of *qi*.

Another use of Even technique is for treatment of trauma. The impact of physical injury, such as a fall or an auto accident, damages the flow of *sanjiao qi* (whole body *qi*) as the impelling force from the trauma travels from the exterior of the body to the interior. An important aspect of treatment in such cases is restoration of normal circulation of the *sanjiao qi*. In addition, treatment should be mild since trauma patients are in a weakened condition. The therapeutic requirements of treatment for trauma are best met by light Even technique, due to its ability to move the *qi* by means of mild stimulation.

Consider the case of a young woman who came for treatment about two hours after an auto accident. The accident was so serious that the steering wheel of the patient's car was bent from impact with her chest. The patient was taken by ambulance directly to a hospital's emergency room, but was released when it was determined she had suffered no injury or bleeding. Upon her release from the hospital, the patient immediately sought acupuncture treatment.

In addition to feeling "beat up all over," the patient complained that her sense of reality was altered in that her mental and emotional being seemed to have no connection with her body. Her pulses were deep, thin, and rapid. Pulses in both *cun* positions were weak. A basic prescription for trauma was followed, using the points Ren 6 *Qihai*, Sanjiao 5 *Waiguan*, and Stomach 36 *Zusanli*.

Treatment began with insertion of needles in the Yang to Yin sequence, starting with Ren 6 *Qihai* ("Sea of Qi"). From its name, we know that *Qihai* is a very good point for *qi*. This point was so named because, when it is stimulated, the *qi* sensation travels out ("like waves on the sea") rather than in a straight line along the meridian as it does with most other acupuncture points. After the arrival of *qi*, the needle at *Qihai* was gently rotated until the patient had a mild feeling of *qi* spreading across the upper and lower abdomen.

Needles were next inserted bilaterally at Sanjiao 5 *Waiguan*. Bilateral insertion was to create the Even Form of acupuncture prescription, used for its ability to balance and regulate the whole body *qi*. After *de qi* was obtained at each point, needles were rotated very mildly as they were inserted deeply to the other side of the forearm (Through and Through Puncturing), into the area of Pericardium 6 *Neiguan*. Qi sensation *(de qi)* from the deep insertion was also obtained at *Neiguan*. To ensure mild stimulation with such deep insertion, needles were fine gauge. Sanjiao 5 *Waiguan* ("Outer Gate") is useful for problems affecting the exterior of the body, and it promotes circulation of *qi* in the channels. *Neiguan* ("Inner Gate"), as its name indicates, is useful for problems which affect the interior of the body. Both of these points help regulate circulation of the *sanjiao qi*.

Finally, needles were inserted bilaterally at Stomach 36 *Zusanli*. After the arrival of *qi,* mild Even technique was applied. *Zusanli,* while it has many uses, is an emergency point for stroke and heart attack, and also treats irregular heartbeat. It is useful in a prescription for treatment of trauma because of its ability in emergency situations to readjust *qi* ("*qi*" in this context meaning vital function and blood circulation).

Needles were retained for only a short time, from about seven to ten minutes. Even though she still was experiencing discomfort, the patient reported that her pain had lessened with treatment. More significant to the patient was that the feeling of being separated from her body had stopped even before the treatment had ended.

Trauma affects the *qi* of the whole body and, as this prescription of *Qihai, Waiguan,* and *Zusanli* indicates, it takes a number of points to cover the various aspects of bodily *qi.* Equally important is that the treatment itself does not traumatize the patient by being too strong.

Even technique can also be applied for treating neurasthenia, a condition of Excess which becomes one of Deficiency. The combination of excessive physical and mental activity gradually causes depletion, which further leads to an inability to recover with rest and regain a sense of ease. Oddly, the more depleted such patients become, the less ability they have to actually rest, and problems such as restless sleep, insomnia, or mental restlessness can become part of the symptomatic landscape.

Mild Even treatment is useful for treating both the Excess and the Deficient aspects of neurasthenia, and needles are retained for twenty to thirty minutes. By selecting points that have an effect on the nervous system, this kind of treatment causes nerves to repolarize and return to a resting state. According to traditional Chinese medical theory, different internal organs relate to different aspects of the nervous system, so differential diagnosis determines treatment of which organ system is appropriate in each case. One basic prescription for neurasthenia is Ear-*Shenmen*, *Yintang* (Extra Point), Pericardium 6 *Neiguan*, Heart 7 *Shenmen*, and Kidney 3 *Taixi*.

Bu and *Xie* Together

Although most practitioners follow the style of Even technique developed by Yang Ji-Zhou, the influence of Chen Hui on treatment remains. As a result of Chen Hui's explanation—that to *xie* first then *bu*, promotes the presence of normal *qi*—practitioners generally prefer to begin treatment with *xie* technique and finish with *bu*.

Combining *bu* and *xie* techniques in the same treatment is a typical approach for weak patients who have acute conditions, pain, or Excess conditions, such as fever. One main concern when treating patients is their general condition and the strength of treatment they can tolerate. This is even more crucial when treating weak or delicate patients. For example, can a patient who is weak tolerate *xie* technique if that is what the therapy requires?

When treating pain, for example, the usual approach is to treat the pain condition first. Some patients are so weak, however, that no matter what kind of technique is used to treat the pain, some form of *bu* technique must be applied first. This is done to fortify weak patients and enable them to withstand treatment without side effects.

Critical conditions need immediate attention even though patients are weak or delicate. Also, applying *bu* technique first, such as in the case of high fever, would Reinforce rather than Reduce pathogenic factors.

Regardless of whether patients are strong or delicate, *bu* technique is often applied at the end of a Reducing treatment to offset the demands that *xie* technique puts on patients' normal *qi*. Mild moxibustion on Stomach 36 *Zusanli* is frequently used as a method to Reinforce patients at the end of a treatment, or at the beginning or a treatment if necessary.

Following is a brief summary of *bu* and *xie* techniques employed singly and together:

Chart 8-3.

USES OF *BU, XIE,* AND THEIR COMBINATIONS

Absolute *bu*	Weak or delicate patients, Deficiency
Absolute *xie*	Pain, acute conditions, Excess
ping bu ping xie	Even technique
First *xie*, then *bu*	Weak patient with acute, pain, or Excess symptoms
First *bu*, then *xie*	Patient is very weak; *bu* first, then treat acute, pain, or Excess symptoms

Ten Auxiliary Techniques

Move: This technique is used when there is no arrival of *qi*. Without any other movement of the needle, such as lifting and thrusting, the handle of the needle is moved in a circle. The movement of the needle, from its tip to the top of the handle, is in a conical configuration. The size of the circle made by the needle handle should be small, and the strength of the movement mild. The purpose of Move is to induce the arrival of *qi*.

Retreat: One or two minutes before a needle is taken out, it is withdrawn near the body surface and retained for a short while. Then, just before the needle is taken out, *bu* (rotating the needle mildly) or *xie* (rotating the needle strongly) is applied in accordance with the treatment plan.

Forward: Once the needle is inserted and the *qi* still does not arrive, the needle is inserted a little deeper to help induce the arrival of *qi*.

Shaking: As the needle is being withdrawn, it is shaken from front to back, from left to right, or in a circle to enlarge the needle hole and to help the Evil *qi* escape. Shaking is a *xie* (Reducing) technique.

Flick: While a needle is retained it is flicked with a finger to mildly stimulate the acupuncture point. Flick is a *bu* (Reinforcing) technique.

Follow: Gently massaging along a meridian and in the area of an acupuncture point helps to gather *qi* around the point. This may be done before a needle is inserted, and may also be done in the area around a needle once it has been inserted.

Pinch: Pinch is used when the tissue around the needle is too tight to move the needle. Pinching the area around a needle will make the *qi* spread. This softens the area so a needle can be moved. *Xie reducing*

Press: When a needle is inserted and the *qi* has arrived, Press is used when the arrival of *qi* is not ample. The needle is grasped tightly by the index and middle fingers while the thumb presses on the top of the needle handle, in the manner of giving an injection. However, in spite of the pressure applied to the needle, the needle is kept at the same level and is not moved in any way.

Claw: An indentation is made on the acupuncture point with the fingernail of the pressing hand to mark the point's location. In addition, pressing to make the Claw mark causes the *wei qi* to spread and minimizes any damage to the *qi* caused by insertion of the needle.

Cut: At the same time the needle is inserted, the nail of the pressing hand presses ("cuts") to eliminate painful sensation of needle insertion.

Treatments can consist of a single technique or of several techniques together. For example, *Ban Ci* (Half Puncturing), a mild insertion method often used for treating weak or delicate patients, can be followed with Uncover technique when needles are taken out in order to provide a mild form of *xie* (Reducing). Then, moxibustion can be applied to the points that were needled or to Stomach 36 *Zusanli* to Reinforce the patient at the end of treatment. Some practitioners like to use elaborate combinations of techniques. Other practitioners follow an equally eloquent style of treatment, but one that relies on the use of only a few techniques performed with great skill.

9

Dao Qi, A Jewel of the Ancients

The Revival of *Dao Qi*

Although the technique of *Dao Qi* is mentioned in the *Nei Jing*, it was disregarded for nearly two thousand years until the Yuan Dynasty. The first person to emphasize the use of *Dao Qi* was the acupuncturist and herbalist Li Dong-Yuan, who is most famous for his *Treatise on the Spleen and Stomach (Pi Wei Lun)*.

Li Dong-Yuan lived during a time of famine in China, and this greatly influenced his thinking. Since Acquired Essence of food and water *(hou tian zhi jing)*—which maintains the body's vital activities and metabolism—is derived from the functions of the Spleen and Stomach, Li Dong-Yuan emphasized a correlation between good health and the proper workings of the digestive system.

According to the *Ling Shu*, all health disorders are due to disorders in *qi* movement, resulting in some aspect of the bodily *qi* being out of its normal position. *"Dao"* is a verb that means "guide" or "lead," and the technique of *Dao Qi* is to lead *qi* to the problem area. The purpose of *Dao*

Qi is to restore the *qi* of the meridians and of the *zang-fu* (internal organs) to its proper order, and to regulate the movement of *qi*. Li Dong-Yuan held that the technique of *Dao Qi* pertains to the *qi* of the digestive system.

Basic Chinese medical theory maintains that all life phenomena come from the changes and movements of *qi*, and that all the different body functions depend on a healthy Stomach and Spleen to provide them with a constant supply of *qi*.

The *qi* of food essence produced by the Spleen and Stomach becomes *ying qi* (Nutrient *qi*, or Constructive *qi*) and *wei qi* (Defensive *qi*), which are associated as the *qi* of the Middle *jiao*. In addition, *qi* of food essence combines with Clean *qi* inhaled by the Lungs to form the *qi* of the Upper *jiao*, the *zong qi* or Pectoral *qi*, which regulates transportation of *qi* and blood to the whole body. The *qi* of the Lower *jiao* (*yuan qi*, Original *qi*; also called Primary *qi*) stimulates and promotes the functions of the internal organs and their associated tissues. In order to be maintained and not be depleted, the *yuan qi* also needs to be supplemented by the refined essence of food and water produced by the Spleen and Stomach. The *qi* which flows in the meridians (*jing qi*, Meridian *qi*), also known as Vital *qi* (*zhen qi*, or *zheng qi*), is formed from the combined *qi* of the Lower, Middle, and Upper *jiao*.

When the Stomach and Spleen functions are regular, the ascending and descending process of *qi* is normal. The pure, clean *qi* from food essence ascends to the Lungs, from the Lungs goes out to the rest of the body, and then goes down as waste to be eliminated as urine and stool. Good health occurs when the various kinds of *qi* remain in proper order.

Chart 9-1.

CORRESPONDENCES OF *QI* TO ITS
POSITION IN THE BODY

Jiao and Associated *Qi*	*Jiao* Functions	Quality of *Qi* Within Each *Jiao*
Upper *jiao*: zong qi	Respiration and blood circulation	Clean, like a fine mist
Middle *jiao*: zhong qi	Digestion; produces *ying qi* and *wei qi*	Like a froth
Lower *jiao*: yuan qi	Water metabolism; discharge of wastes	Turbid, like a drainage ditch

Irregularities in health arise when overfatigue, poor eating habits, and mental and emotional stress damage the Vital *qi* and deplete the *yuan qi*. This damages the normal flow of *qi* and creates stasis, typified by symptoms ranging from mild discomfort to pain. When the *yuan qi* of the Lower *jiao* is depleted and the body's balance is lost, it also induces the Yin Fire of the Kidney to rise, and with it rises the turbid *qi* of the Lower *jiao*. When the turbid *qi* ascends and does not go down, the clear, clean *qi* may not ascend. If turbid *qi* rises, there can be symptoms of nausea, vomiting, borborygmus, edema, phlegm, or cough; when clear *qi* does not ascend, the sensory orifices are not clear and there can be dizziness. According to Li Dong-Yuan, all of this occurs because the Stomach *qi* is weakened, and then other types of *qi* go out of their normal positions.

Dao Qi is a unique method of regulating *qi* movement and making *qi* go back to its regular place, which promotes quicker response to treatment. In the *Nei Jing, Dao Qi* is described as "from Yang to Yin, and from Yin to

Yang therapy." Li Dong-Yuan explained that *Dao Qi* begins with the arrival of *qi* at the outer level of the body, and then transfers *qi* internally ("from Yang to Yin"). Additionally, *Dao Qi* activates *qi* to come out from deep within the body to promote healing ("from Yin to Yang"). For Li Dong-Yuan, this meant that the effects of *Dao Qi* went from the *wei qi* to the internal body (Yang to Yin), and came out from the depths of the *ying qi* (Yin to Yang). Since the *wei qi* and the *ying qi* are associated with the Middle *jiao*, and therefore with the Stomach and Spleen, Li Dong-Yuan associated *Dao Qi* with the *qi* of the digestive system.

Dao Qi Technique

Needle Insertion and Manipulation

Like other outstanding physicians, Li Dong-Yuan emphasized the coordinated efforts of the needling hand and the pressing hand when inserting needles. First pressing on acupuncture points with the pressing hand and then inserting with the needling hand, or both pressing and inserting simultaneously, decreases the sensation of needle insertion. It also promotes better needling reaction *(de qi)*. Lack of needling reaction indicates poor quality technique, poor point location, or a patient too weak to respond to the use of needles. By obtaining the arrival of *qi*, a practitioner begins to generate an ample supply of *qi* to send to the problem area.

After *de qi* is obtained, *Dao Qi* begins with thrusting and lifting of the needle repeatedly, usually for a period of three to four minutes each time a needle is manipulated. A three-minute to four-minute application of *Dao Qi* technique is called "one performance" *("yi du")*. For patients who are weak or who are sensitive to needling, the duration of a performance of *Dao Qi* can be reduced. The speed of lifting and thrusting is always the same in both directions. The depth to which a needle is inserted and the level to which it is lifted should never change, but should remain the same throughout repeated lifting and thrusting. Rotation of the needle is neither too fast nor too slow, and always with even stimulus, even speed, and equal-sized turns in both directions. Needles are aimed in the direction of the problem being treated, and the angle of insertion should remain the same throughout the treatment.

Every aspect of needle manipulation for *Dao Qi* should remain the same—speed of thrusting, lifting, and rotation; depth of thrusting and lifting; stimulus of treatment; and so forth. The entire time that needles are manipulated, the practitioner's mind must be only on making the *qi* run and on where the *qi* must go. Even the most brief lapse of attention on the part of the practitioner can break the effect of *Dao Qi*. A beneficial side effect of this technique is that the presence of mind and the precise details of needle manipulation required to perform *Dao Qi* raise the practitioner's overall level of technical skill.

For *Dao Qi* to be most effective, the patient needs to be calm. When the patient is relaxed it is easier for the practitioner to get the effect of *Dao Qi*. Furthermore, if the patient is calm and can clearly report the sensations resulting from treatment, it is easier for the practitioner to control what is happening. *Dao Qi* is very much a cooperative effort between patient and practitioner.

In addition to a sensation of heaviness or soreness at the needle site resulting from *de qi*, the patient should feel *qi* running in the direction which the practitioner intends. The sensation of *Dao Qi* is different from that of any other technique and feels to the patient like a constant flow of water or air, a feeling described in the *Nei Jing* as "light and wonderful." The most ideal feeling is one that runs all the way to the area being treated. That may happen the first time *Dao Qi* is performed in a treatment, or the distance that the feeling reaches may be slight and only gradually increase with successive applications of *Dao Qi* during a treatment.

The flowing feeling of *Dao Qi* should continue for some time after needle manipulation has ceased. The amount of time the feeling continues can be as short as a few minutes, or can last the entire length of a treatment with only one performance of *Dao Qi*. Some patients have reported the feeling of *Dao Qi* lasting for a few days after treatment. Any time during treatment that the patient begins to lose the feeling of *qi* constantly flowing, *Dao Qi* needs to be repeated.

Some practitioners have the notion that any time *qi* runs along the meridian, it is *Dao Qi*. The sensation of *qi* moving along the meridian can occur when there is a strong arrival of *qi (de qi)*. It can occur when a practitioner increases the strength of needle manipulation being applied. *Qi* moving along the meridian can also occur, as we have already seen, with the use of Even technique when treating pain. None of these is *Dao Qi*. The hallmark of *Dao Qi* is its distinctive method of needle manipulation and the unique feeling of *qi* constantly flowing like water from the acupuncture point to the problem area.

Strength of Treatment

of treatment should not be taken to mean strength of stimulus a light, constant sensation. Rather, strength corresponds to tion of *Dao Qi* in a treatment, and to the duration of a treatment. The number of times that *Dao Qi* is performed and the total time of treatment are determined primarily by the condition being treated and by the length of treatment which the patient can tolerate. *Dao Qi* is repeated more times for treatment of pain, which, in effect, lengthens the time of a treatment. Weak patients generally cannot tolerate *Dao Qi* repeated too many times, which shortens the total treatment time. Another method of providing lighter treatment for weak patients is to use finer gauge needles.

How to Choose Points

Choice of acupuncture points for *Dao Qi* is according to basic *Nei Jing* theory of point selection. For treatment of the internal organs, "If Yin is diseased then treat Yang; if Yang is diseased then treat Yin." This means selecting Back-*Shu* Points for treatment of the Yin organs and Front-*Mu* Points for the Yang organs. Remote Points prescribed by the *Nei Jing* for treatment of the internal organs are *Yuan* (Source) Points for the *zang*, and *He*-Sea Points and Inferior *He*-Sea Points for the *fu*. There is a general preference for the use of Remote Points since they are more conducive to safe manipulation of needles. More importantly, Remote Points are generally considered the most powerful of all the acupuncture points.

The *Nei Jing* recommends *Ying*-Spring Points for treatment of problems affecting skin or muscles, and *Shu*-Stream Points for conditions involving the muscles or the meridians. Frequently, *Shu*-Stream Points are used as a substitute for *Ying*-Spring Points since the *Ying*-Spring Points are more painful to treat.

A few acupuncture points selected for *Dao Qi* have been found through experience to be more effective than *Ying*-Spring Points and *Shu*-Stream

Points. Pericardium 7 *Daling* is a very useful point, but it is also extremely painful when needled. Even though *Daling* in theory is the recommended point for *Dao Qi*, Pericardium 6 *Neiguan* is used instead. Not only is *Neiguan* less painful, it is a more powerful and effective point than *Daling*. Another substitute found to be more effective is Spleen 6 *Sanyinjiao,* used instead of Spleen 3 *Taibai*. Occasionally, points local to the problem as well as other Remote points—such as *Xi* (Cleft) Points—are also used, but this is not typical of *Dao Qi* therapy.

Chart 9-2.

SELECTION OF POINTS FOR *DAO QI*

Area Treated:	Acupuncture Point:
Skin, muscles	*Ying*-Spring Points
Muscles, meridians	*Shu*-Stream Points
Yang organs (*fu*)	Front-*Mu* Points
	He-Sea Points
Yin organs (*zang*)	Back-*Shu* Points
	Yuan (Source) Points

Depth of Insertion

How deeply needles can be inserted is determined by two main factors. First is the location of the acupuncture points. Areas that are more muscular can be needled deeper, while insertion in bony areas has to be more shallow.

The other determining factor is the location of the condition being treated. For problems affecting skin or muscles, the insertion is very shallow.

Insertion for treatment of the Yang organs (*fu*) is a little deeper than that for skin, muscles, or meridians. The deepest insertion is for treatment of the Yin organs *(zang)* and for treatment of chronic conditions.

Placement of Needles

One question regarding treatment that acupuncturists face is whether to place needles on the same side of the body as the location of the condition, or whether to place needles on the side opposite the condition. There are two simple guidelines for placement of needles in relation to the location of the health problem. These guidelines apply not only to *Dao Qi* but also to acupuncture treatment in general.

When an acute health problem has not yet manifested in the pulses, it indicates the pathogenic factors are still at the most superficial level. In such cases, balance is restored by treating the side opposite the condition.

When treating chronic conditions, if treatment of the affected side is not providing results then treatment is switched to the opposite side of the body. This is done because the lack of results shows that the affected side has an insufficient amount of *qi* to provide a response to treatment.

Dao Qi Compared to *Bu, Xie,* and Even Technique

Dao Qi, bu, and *xie* all employ lifting, thrusting, and rotating of needles. *Bu* technique is accomplished by slow thrusting and quick lifting of needles. Or, *bu* is performed with greater stimulus when thrusting and lighter stimulus when lifting. Another *bu* technique is Three Levels Down. *Xie* technique is just the opposite of *bu* in all of these examples. *Dao Qi*, in contrast, must always be executed with the same speed of thrusting and lifting, the same degree of stimulus, and even amplitude of rotation.

From the first step to the last, all aspects of needle movement for *Dao Qi* are constant.

The purpose of *bu* technique is to add to a Deficiency of Vital *qi*, while *xie* takes away the Excess of pathogenic *qi*. There are different explanations for Even technique. The most famous is from Chen Hui, who said that health problems arise because Evil *qi* enters the body and weakens the Vital *qi*. According to Chen Hui, the purpose of Even technique is first to push out Evil *qi* and then to fortify the normal *qi*. Even though Yang Ji-Zhou revolutionized the application of Even technique, its basic function and purpose remain unchanged. The purpose of *Dao Qi* is different from those of *bu*, *xie*, or Even techniques. *Dao Qi* leads *qi* to the problem area so as to restore the *qi* to its normal order and promote its normal circulation.

If *Dao Qi* were added to the list of techniques in chart 8-3 from Chapter 8, all the various acupuncture techniques could be categorized as follows:

> Absolute *bu*
>
> Absolute *xie*
>
> Even *(ping bu ping xie)*
>
> First *xie,* then *bu*
>
> First *bu,* then *xie*
>
> "None of the above" *(Dao Qi)*

Examples of Treatment with *Dao Qi*

The first two examples of treatment with *Dao Qi* deal with diseases caused by disorders of *qi* in the Upper and Middle *jiao*, leading to an attack by the rising of the Yin Fire of the Kidney. This condition is called in Chinese "shen huo pian kang." "Shen huo" is the Fire of the Kidney. "Pian" means "irregular" (i.e., "unhealthy"). "Kang" means "flare up" into a burst of flame.

I. Stress, Insomnia, Depression

The patient continually experienced stress at work and usually had restless sleep. He started having palpitations at night and was becoming unable to concentrate. He experienced no joy in any aspect of his life and he felt worried all the time, though he had no reasons for the cause of the worry. The patient was usually tired and weak, and had no appetite.

The patient's pulses were thready and rapid. The tip of his tongue was red, and the tongue coating was very thin.

Diagnosis was that weakness of the Heart and the Spleen induced rising of the Kidney Fire, which attacked the Ministerial Fire of the Heart (jun huo). The combination of stress and the hyperactivity of the Ministerial Fire created stasis of qi, manifesting as a kind of depression. Acupuncture points selected to strengthen functions of the Heart and Spleen, and to lead the Yin Fire of the Kidney back to its place in the Lower jiao, were Pericardium 6 Neiguan, Heart 7 Shenmen, and Spleen 6 Sanyinjiao. Since the patient's condition was severe, all points were needled bilaterally.

Dao Qi was performed on all the acupuncture points in succession from Yang to Yin. Once Dao Qi was flowing from all the points simultaneously, the needles were retained for thirty minutes more. During the treatment, the patient's pulses returned to normal, and when he returned for the second treatment all his symptoms were gone.

II. Cough, Shortness of Breath

The patient was very thin, had poor appetite, and was often tired due to overwork. He suddenly developed a sore throat, difficulty swallowing, shortness of breath, and a dry cough. With the acute symptoms came an insatiable thirst which was worse at night, a tight feeling in the chest, and insomnia. The patient also reported a feverish sensation in the palms of the hands and the soles of the feet.

Examination of the throat showed no swelling or redness. Pulses were thready and rapid. The whole tongue was red, and the tongue coating was thin and yellowish brown.

Diagnostic conclusions were that weakness of the Stomach *qi* permitted the Fire of the Kidney to rise and attack the Lungs. Acupuncture points selected for *Dao Qi* were Lung 9 *Taiyuan* and Kidney 3 *Taxi* with the goal of balancing the functions of the Lung and Kidney.

Needles were first inserted bilaterally in Lung 9 *Taiyuan*. After needling sensation *(de qi)* was obtained in both *Taiyuan* points, a needle was inserted into Kidney 3 *Taixi*, and *Dao Qi* was applied. Then, a needle was inserted into *Taixi* on the other side and again *Dao Qi* was applied to the point. The sensation of *Dao Qi* ran up to the throat and the patient reported feeling not so thirsty and dry. When the feeling of *qi* flowing at *Taixi* began to diminish, *Dao Qi* was repeated a second time.

When the patient returned he said that he had slept well the night after the treatment, the feeling in the chest had become normal, and there was no cough, although his throat was still a little sore. After the second treatment the remaining symptoms improved, but not completely. After five treatments all the symptoms were gone and never returned.

This patient illustrates that *Dao Qi* need not be applied to all the acupuncture points used in a treatment. Although Lung 9 *Taiyuan* is in a bony area, what limits the amount of needle manipulation is that *Taiyuan* is next to the radial artery. The example for the treatment of trigeminal neuralgia, which follows later, will show the use of *Dao Qi* at acupuncture points located in bony areas.

III. Diarrhea

Due to overeating, and to eating a large amount of rich foods, the patient developed watery diarrhea, intestinal gas, Stomach pain, and loss of appetite. When the patient came for treatment, he had been suffering the symptoms for three days.

The patient felt tired and had a dull appearance. His pulses were slow and wiry, the tip of his tongue was slightly red, and the tongue coating was thin, greasy, and a little yellow.

Acupuncture points selected to regulate the *qi* in the Stomach and the intestines were Ren 12 *Zhongwan* and Stomach 36 *Zusanli*. Selection of points was based on the *Nei Jing* theory, "When Yang is diseased, treat Yin." *Zhongwan* is the Front-*Mu* Point of the Stomach, as well as the Influential Point for the Yang organs *(fu)*. *Mu* Points are considered Yin because of their location in Yin areas of the torso. *Zusanli* is the *He*-Sea Point of the Stomach and it is in the lower extremities, also a Yin location. When there is diarrhea, Stomach 36 is one of the most important points to consider for treatment.

Dao Qi from *Zhongwan* reached about two inches below the navel. Then, *Dao Qi* was applied at *Zhongwan* to direct the *qi* up into the Stomach. Since symptoms were in both the intestines and the Stomach, *Dao Qi* at

Zhongwan was directed to treat both areas. *Dao Qi* was directed down to the intestines first because rising of the turbid *qi* blocked normal, clean *qi* from ascending to the Stomach. Sending the dirty *qi* down first ensured that the normal *qi* could go up to its place in the Stomach. Finally, *Dao Qi* was applied to *Zusanli* on both legs, with the sensation running all the way to the Stomach. In any treatment with *Dao Qi*, the further the sensation travels, the better the effect.

The last two examples deal with treatment of disorders of *qi* in the meridians. These are problems on the surface of the body, not internal problems.

IV. Trigeminal Neuralgia

This patient came for treatment of a sudden onset of pain that was in the zygomatic area, and around the mouth and chin. The patient's level of pain was extreme, and the skin in the affected area was painful when touched.

She had experienced previous attacks of pain which had become progressively severe with each episode. At first she thought the pain was due to a toothache that was getting worse, but examination by a dentist proved negative.

During the diagnosis, questioning revealed that her symptoms always coincided with overwork and fatigue. Her pulses were rapid and tight, and her tongue was red with a very thin tongue coat. She was diagnosed as having trigeminal neuralgia caused by Yin (i.e., Kidney) Fire and turbid *qi* attacking the head.

Points selected for treatment were Stomach 7 *Xiaguan*, Large Intestine 3 *Sanjian*, and Urinary Bladder 65 *Shugu*, with the goal of sending the dirty *qi* back to its place in the Lower *jiao*, and regulating the *qi* in the face.

Treatment began at Stomach 7 *Xiaguan*, with the *qi* sensation running from *Xiaguan* to the lower jaw and to the mouth. *Dao Qi* was performed at *Xiaguan* three times, and then at Large Intestine 3 *Sanjian* three times. *Sanjian* was inserted on the side opposite that of the facial pain. Finally, *Dao Qi* was performed at *Shugu* three times, causing the *qi* sensation to run up the leg. *Shugu* and *Sanjian* are very sensitive points. The length of time that *Dao Qi* is performed at such points may need to be abbreviated in order to prevent treatment from being too strong for the patient.

Some reduction in pain was obtained during the first treatment. After three treatments there was complete recovery. This case is unusual since trigeminal neuralgia is a stubborn condition which often requires many treatments. The patient's speedy recovery is due to more than one factor. *Dao Qi* itself should hasten the regular response. In addition, clinical experience has shown that treatments for pain are most successful if treatment is given when pain is actually present, rather than between pain attacks.

V. *Bi* Syndrome, Shoulder Pain

After straining his right shoulder at work, the patient would intermittently suffer pain when lifting, but not at other times. The patient sought treatment because the condition had become chronic. The shoulder pain, which was in the area of the Small Intestine Channel, was aggravated by pressing though there was no swelling or signs of inflammation. Pain on lifting was more severe when the patient was overtired from work. His pulses were wiry and slow; the tongue coating was thin and yellow, and the tongue body was a normal color.

The diagnosis was that the Constructive *qi* and the Defensive *qi* in the area of the shoulder were in disorder, allowing Wind, Cold, and Damp to enter and block the normal flow of the meridian.

In order to Reduce the external pathogenic factors of Wind, Cold, and Damp, the affected area was tapped with a Cutaneous hammer to the point of appearance of petechiae but not to the point of bleeding. Then the shoulder was cupped. The entire procedure of Reducing took about ten minutes. After the cups were removed, Reinforcing with indirect moxibustion was applied to the shoulder area for about five minutes.

Upon completion of both *xie* (Reducing) and *bu* (Reinforcing) of the affected area, *Dao Qi* was applied to Gall Bladder 34 *Yanglingquan* on the left side. For chronic conditions, the first treatment is commonly on the side opposite the problem. This is done because the unaffected side has more normal *qi* than the affected side.

Dao Qi was performed four times in a twenty-minute period and only *Yanglingquan* on the left side was used. The patient felt about ninety percent recovered at the end of the treatment and when he returned for a second treatment he was pain free.

There are a number of reasons why this treatment with only one acupuncture point was so successful. First, the effectiveness of the *Dao Qi* was enhanced by beginning the treatment with Cutaneous tapping, cupping, and moxibustion in order to Reduce pathogenic factors and to Reinforce the *qi* in the affected area.

Second, the approach chosen for treatment called for selection of an acupuncture point on the side opposite the problem. The use of *Yanglingquan* on the side opposite the problem, through experience, has been established to be efficacious for treatment of pain and motor problems in the shoulder.

Third, *Yanglingquan* is a Remote Point. Characteristic of the classical style of acupuncture is a strong preference for the use of Remote Points. *Nei Jing* theory considers Remote Points generally the most effective of all the acupuncture points, and clinical experience over the long history of Chinese medicine verifies the significant effectiveness of Remote Points.

Finally, *Yanglingquan* is the Influential Point for tendons, which regulate movement. Any problem associated with movement, whether it is limited movement or whether it is due to injury as a result of movement, indicates involvement of tendons. Treatment with *Yanglingquan* for tendon-related problems is most effective when the affected area, in this case the shoulder, is moved at the same time the needle is being manipulated.

10

Moxibustion

The Miracle Drug, *Artemisia Vulgaris*

The word for "acupuncture" in Chinese *("zhen jiu")* includes both needles *(zhen)* and moxibustion *(jiu)*. In the West far more emphasis is placed on the use of needles, while the significant and extensive therapeutic value of moxibustion is often overlooked.

Clinical experiences over the centuries have shown that in cases when the use of needles or herbs is not successful, moxibustion can still provide therapeutic results. The use of moxa on the navel is especially good for treating intractable or lingering health problems. In conditions of collapse, such as Deficient type stroke, moxibustion can be a life-saving therapy. One treatment for life-threatening collapse is a tea brewed from high-grade wild Chinese ginseng *(shan shen)*. However, a single root of good quality wild ginseng can easily cost tens of thousands of dollars. Moxibustion on Ren 8 *Shenque*, Ren 6 *Qihai*, and Ren 4 *Guanyuan* can have the same effects as the wild ginseng for treatment of collapse, while costing only a few cents.

Not only is moxibustion an effective form of treatment, it is important for preventative purposes and is a superb method of raising the body's resistance. Zhuang Zi, the great Daoist philosopher of the Warring States Period and student of Lao Zi, wrote that Confucius had exceptionally robust health and never got ill because of his regular use of moxibustion.

The Chinese word for moxibustion therapy, *"jiu,"* is a compound character from two words: "time" and "fire." Making use of heat by sitting close to a fire was an early form of therapy for various afflictions due to attack from external pathogenic factors, such as Wind, Cold, or Damp. Moxa therapy first developed from experiments with the smoldering twigs of various plants to compare their therapeutic effectiveness. These experiments led to expanded understanding of moxibustion's use as a treatment modality, and created a variety of moxa therapies that are more elaborate in China than those presently used in the West. One example is the use of pastes made from various herbs. The paste is made into a two-millimeter-thick patty and placed directly on acupuncture points, with different herb pastes selected for different effects. Then, a smoldering moxa cone is placed on the herb paste.

China's northern climate promotes more emphasis on moxa therapy than does the climate of the south, resulting in a more developed approach to moxibustion among northern physicians. There have always been some northern practitioners who never use needles or herbs for treatment, only moxa therapy, and it is possible to still find a few such physicians in practice.

In the process of experimenting with various herbs for moxibustion, the discovery of *Artemisia vulgaris* (mugwort, *ai rong*) led to its use as the primary herb for moxa therapy because of the unique ability of its heat to penetrate deeply beneath the skin. Even in China, moxa therapy is generally taken to mean the therapeutic effect of applying ignited mugwort over affected parts of the body and to acupuncture points. Though other herbs are sometimes combined with mugwort, the discussion here of moxibustion will be only in reference to the use of *Artemisia vulgaris*.

A sign of good health is normal circulation of *qi* and blood, and mugwort is therapeutically effective because the heat of the smoldering herb penetrates deeply into the body, stimulating the circulation of *qi* and blood in the meridians. In addition, the volatile oils of the burning moxa penetrate into the skin and the meridians, and have a therapeutic effect as well. Point location is not as critical as with needle insertion because heat from the moxa emanates into a relatively large area.

The older and drier the moxa, the better its effects. Moxa for clinical use should be at least three years old, while good quality moxa is aged seven years or more. The more chronic the ailment or the more severe the disease condition that is being treated, the older the moxa should be, in order to get the best possible results.

Often, the effects of moxibustion on acupuncture points are identical to those from the insertion of needles. Stomach 36 *Zusanli* is an excellent point for treating shortness of breath; moxibustion or acupuncture on *Zusanli* are equally effective. Sometimes, only needle insertion will produce a desired effect, as when *Zusanli* is used as an emergency point for heart attack. Other times, moxibustion provides superior effects. The *Nei Jing* recommends regular application of moxibustion on *Zusanli* as the premier method of promoting longevity and good health. Part of any practitioner's expanding clinical repertoire is knowledge of the effects that various methods of applying treatment can have on acupuncture points.

There are many methods of applying moxa, but they can be reduced to two categories: 1) direct, which is the placement of ignited mugwort directly on the patient's skin; and 2) indirect, which consists of various methods of warming and stimulating the meridians without the smoldering moxa coming into direct contact with the patient's skin. Currently, indirect moxibustion is used more frequently because it is safer and more comfortable for the patient.

In many instances the effects from the different ways of applying moxibustion are the same, though with many of the classical moxa prescriptions, direct moxibustion is often the intended method. When the *Nei Jing* recommends frequent moxibustion on Stomach 36 *Zusanli*, it says, "*Zusanli* should never be dry," an allusion to the inevitable, though occasional, small water blisters resulting from frequent direct moxibustion. At times, only a specific way of applying moxa will get the desired results. Indirect moxibustion on salt, garlic, ginger, or herb pastes is selected according to the effect that each procedure produces. Direct moxibustion is the preferred method of treatment on Stomach 36 *Zusanli* and Gall Bladder 39 *Xuanzhong* for preventing stroke. The use of direct moxibustion has an added effect that other methods of moxibustion lack: it removes pathogenic *qi* from the acupuncture points and meridians. As a prophylactic for stroke, direct moxibustion Reduces pathogenic Wind from the Channels and Collaterals, as well as helps to Reinforce and circulate the Vital *qi*.

Moxa therapy is often a welcome form of treatment for patients because the effects of moxibustion are both vitalizing and relaxing.

Moxibustion mildly stimulates the circulation of *qi* and blood, which improves the metabolism and gives a sense of wellness, while the gentle warmth of moxa is very comforting.

Moxibustion can also be used to promote emotional balance by strengthening general health. In Chinese medicine, mental and emotional health have an important reciprocal relationship with health in general. Unbalanced emotions and emotional upset—known as "internal causes of disease"—reduce the normal flow of *qi* and blood to the tissues. On the other hand, according to the *Nei Jing*, people who are healthy have the strength to control their emotions, which enables them to make themselves happy and kind. Basic Chinese medical theory holds that different aspects of the consciousness come out of different organ functions, rather than from the brain alone. When the health of the internal organs is strong, then there is a corresponding mental and emotional well-being. Conversely, people who are weak can be very emotional because they are not strong enough to control their emotions. Moxibustion on *Qihai* Ren 6 is a simple and effective prescription for promoting emotional stability, resulting from the ability of *Qihai* to fortify and to promote circulation of the Vital *qi*.

The scope of moxa therapy can be as comprehensive as that of herbal therapy or acupuncture. As we have seen, some physicians practice moxibustion to the exclusion of all other therapies. One indication of the effectiveness of moxa is that when other therapies are unable to get any improvement, moxibustion can still get results. However, rather than wait for the progress of treatment to reach such a stalemate, moxibustion can be combined initially with other treatment modalities to enhance the therapeutic response.

Guidelines for Treatment with Moxa

Moxibustion is best known for treating Cold, Deficient, and chronic conditions. Yet, the use of moxa is not only for Cold problems but also for Yang and Heat problems. Acute conditions are Yang, and moxibustion is used for treating acute conditions such as diarrhea, influenza, and the common cold. Moxibustion may even be used for treating febrile conditions resulting from exogenous pathogenic factors if the fever is not too high. Mild moxibustion combined with acupuncture at Du 14 *Dazhui*, a point famous for treating fever, spreads away the Evil *qi* inducing the fever. Pathogenic *qi* tends to stagnate, while normal *qi* circulates. The heat of moxibustion induces circulation of pathogenic *qi*, causing it to disperse. Moxibustion may also be combined with needle insertion for treatment of Excess type stroke and for convulsion. Reducing (*xie*) treatment with needles for these Yang conditions is followed by mild moxibustion on the navel after *xie* technique has Reduced the Excess of pathogenic factors. This is done because the disease condition results in a weakening of the patient's normal *qi*, and mild moxibustion helps Reinforce the patient.

As with the insertion of acupuncture needles, moxibustion is applied to the body in a certain sequence, namely from Yang to Yin. This means treating points on the back side before the front, and proceeding from top to bottom, meaning from the head to the torso, to the arms, and then to the legs.

Reinforcing and Reducing techniques are possible with moxibustion, and the general rule is that *xie* (Reducing) is treatment for a longer time, and that *bu* (Reinforcing) is treatment for a shorter time. With moxibustion, as with acupuncture, time as a determining factor for *bu* and *xie* is flexible. Deep level Cold may require application of moxa for a long time. Moxibustion on Gall Bladder 39 *Xuanzhong* for treating weak patients who complain of being "cold to the bone" may be for a minimum of fifteen minutes per acupuncture point when using moxa-stick. Care must be taken not to damage the skin when applying moxa for a long time. Warming-needle technique using smoldering moxa on needle handles to treat Cold conditions is usually performed for at least twenty minutes. Another means of determining *bu* and *xie* is the strength of the treatment, with mild moxibustion resulting in *bu* and strong moxa treatment resulting in *xie*.

Generally, moxa treatments employ three to five moxa cones for each acupuncture point, or ten to fifteen minutes of moxa-stick. The size or number of moxa cones used for treatment, the duration of treatment with warming needle and with moxa-stick application, and the number of points selected for treatment, are partly determined by the patient's general constitution. The most important constitutional factor is the patient's general strength. For a weakened patient, treatment that is too long or too strong can further weaken the patient and aggravate the patient's symptoms. The second constitutional factor is the patient's age, with the elderly, children, and infants considered the most delicate.

The nature of the pathological condition also affects the duration and strength of treatment. Application of moxa for Cold conditions can extend treatment for a longer time and still not have a Reducing effect on the patient's *qi*. Finally, the site where moxibustion is applied has a bearing on treatment, since the skin in some areas of the body is more delicate and sensitive to heat than in other areas. Special attention is also given to avoid burning patients when either direct or indirect moxibustion is applied to areas with reduced feeling due to conditions such as numbness or neuropathy.

Caution is advised when considering moxibustion for patients with Yin *xu* (Yin Deficiency) or with high blood pressure. Moxa for these kinds of patients is prohibited in the areas of the head, torso, and upper extremities, because heat from the moxa can make these conditions worse. In the case of high blood pressure, moxibustion in the contraindicated areas can make the blood pressure higher or can cause a stroke. However, points below the knees may be used, such as Stomach 36 *Zusanli* and Gall Bladder 39 *Xuanzhong* for high blood pressure, and mild, indirect moxibustion on ginger on Kidney 3 *Taixi* in cases of Yin *xu*.

The use of moxibustion is strictly contraindicated when the patient has high fever, due either to exogenous factors or to Deficiency of Yin. Additionally, moxa is not used over the Heart or the Liver, near arteries, on the neck or face, or on the abdomen and lumbosacral area of pregnant women.

General rules for applying moxa can be flexible. Even the *Nei Jing* guideline for treatment—"For Excess use more needles and less moxa; for Deficiency use fewer needles and more moxa"—is not a hard and fast rule. Factors determining the approach to moxa treatment are whether the patient is strong or weak; whether the pathological condition is acute or chronic, Excess or Deficient; and whether there is pain or no pain.

Moxibustion Prescriptions

A Method of Treating According to Meridian Theory

One use of acupuncture and moxibustion is for cosmetics and for facelift. In modern times this is usually done only to improve the physical appearance. In ancient times, more emphasis was placed on the relationship of physical appearance with underlying health, and physiognomy was used as one aspect of diagnosis for determining the patient's health condition and developing a corresponding treatment plan. Historically, this particular approach to meridian theory combined with moxa therapy has placed emphasis on the Kidney and the Liver meridians as most important.

The meridian indications listed below are according to relationships of eight select meridians to different body types and to various cosmetic imbalances. By following these correspondences, moxibustion can be applied to the appropriate meridians in order to enhance the overall effects of therapy. Treating this way with moxibustion need not necessarily be on specific acupuncture points, and can be anywhere along a meridian. Ancient practitioners had a more expanded view of meridian theory: they considered the meridians which travel from Back-*Shu* Points to their related organs as part of the Regular Channel of its corresponding organ. For example, moxibustion on Urinary Bladder 22 *Sanjiaoshu* is considered a method of applying moxa to the Sanjiao Channel.

Liver Channel: The Liver is known as the "blood bank." It stores blood and regulates the volume of circulating blood. The Liver also governs the smooth flow of qi and therefore promotes the smooth functioning of the Channels and Collaterals and of the zang-fu, especially digestion and absorption by the Spleen and Stomach. Smooth flow of qi also relates to healthy emotional activity, and Liver dysfunction may be accompanied by emotional imbalances such as depression, irritability, or uncontrolled anger.

Moxa on the Liver Channel is selected for overweight and obese patients, and for freckling, rashes on the face, and dark spotting of the skin such as seen with Addison's Disease.

Kidney Channel: The Kidney is the "Root of *qi*" for the entire body, and is the source of the body's Yin and Yang.

Moxibustion on the Kidney Channel is for the very lean ("bony") type. Other indications that correspond to the Kidney Channel are swelling or edema, and oily skin. Freckling of the skin is due to disorder of Kidney function if the patient is also thin. The Kidney is responsible for the production of marrow. The brain is known as the "Sea of marrow" and moxibustion on the Kidney Channel is used for patients with mental or emotional imbalances.

Urinary Bladder Channel: The Urinary Bladder Channel is used to control obesity. Moxa on the Urinary Bladder Channel is for the patient whose face is always red or flushed, as well as for the patient whose face is pale. This channel is for treatment of herpes or rashes on the face that appear before menses, and for menstrual cramping. When freckling appears during pregnancy or postpartum, moxibustion may be applied to the Urinary Bladder Channel.

Generally, the best area for moxibustion on the Urinary Bladder Channel is on the Back-*Shu* Points.

Large Intestine and Small Intestine Channels: The Large Intestine and Small Intestine Channels treat and prevent urticaria, eczema, allergies, constipation, and diarrhea. Moxibustion on these channels is selected for the bony type, and is used to promote weight gain. It is also used to promote skin luster.

Stomach Channel: Moxa on the Stomach Channel increases resistance and prevents the outbreak of herpes and rashes. Moxibustion on the Stomach Channel is used to treat abnormal skin secretions considered to be due to poorly digested food, and improves the color and luster of the skin.

Sanjiao Channel: Moxibustion on the Sanjiao Channel strengthens the *wei qi* (Defensive *qi*). The Sanjiao Channel is selected to stop suppuration of herpes.

Spleen Channel: Spleen functions produce blood and *qi*. The Spleen controls the thickness and the strength of the muscles and gives balance to the musculature.

Twelve Points that Affect the Entire Body

Many acupuncture points treat only their related meridian and organ, not the whole body. Even some important and powerful points, such as *Xi* (Cleft) Points, are selected for their limited effects rather than for treating complex interconnected body systems. The twelve acupuncture points listed below are among those most frequently used with moxa therapy to treat the entire body via their ability to strengthen the metabolism and the body's resistance:

Large Intestine 11 *Quchi*	Ren 4 *Guanyuan*
Stomach 36 *Zusanli*	Urinary Bladder 12 *Fengmen*
Spleen 6 *Sanyinjiao*	Urinary Bladder 13 *Feishu*
Spleen 10 *Xuehai*	Urinary Bladder 18 *Ganshu*
Ren 12 *Zhongwan*	Urinary Bladder 20 *Pishu*
Ren 6 *Qihai*	Urinary Bladder 23 *Shenshu*

These twelve points are well known for their various effects on the whole body metabolism, summarized under the general functions of the production and circulation of *qi* and blood. In addition to these whole body metabolic functions of *qi* and blood, three points—Urinary Bladder 23 *Shenshu*, Spleen 10 *Xuehai*, and Spleen 6 *Sanyinjiao*—govern aspects of the metabolism that Western medicine would define as the endocrine system.

Frequent moxibustion on Urinary Bladder 12 *Fengmen* and Stomach 36 *Zusanli* bolsters the Defensive *qi*, and is a prophylactic treatment for resistance to attack from external pathogenic factors. "*Fengmen*" means "the door to (treating) Wind." The word "Wind" is synonymous with "disease," indicating that *Fengmen* is important for raising the body's resistance to disease.

Miscellaneous Moxa Prescriptions and Examples of Treatment

Shock or collapse, with hands and feet extremely cold, and no pulse or very dim pulse: Ten rice-grain-size moxa cones bilaterally on Kidney 3 *Taixi*.

Irregular heartbeat: Du 4 *Mingmen* and Ren 4 *Guanyuan*. One such patient, age 63, was given this treatment for fifty days, and the pulse returned to completely normal in that time.

Chronic, severe menstrual cramping: The patient's condition grew progressively worse over a five-year period. Seven to nine moxa cones on Ren 4 *Guanyuan*, and on Stomach 28 *Shuidao* bilaterally, were applied once every other day. After one month, the symptoms were greatly improved and treatment was then applied by using moxa-stick.

Cold hands and feet, possibly including stiffness and numbness: Spleen 6 *Sanyinjiao*.

Pulmonary tuberculosis: Urinary Bladder 43 *Gaohuangshu*, Urinary Bladder 17 *Geshu*, and Urinary Bladder 19 *Danshu*. *Gaohuangshu* is not only a point for treating Lung problems, it is a very good moxa point for strengthening immunity.

Tuberculosis is considered a consumptive disease, and characteristic of consumptive diseases is some degree of Yin *xu*. However, in nearly ninety percent of tuberculosis cases, the patient has a white tongue coat, indicating the presence of Cold. If pulses are rapid and weak but the patient's hands and feet are cold, or if the tongue body or tongue coat indicate Cold signs, moxibustion can be used. When determining Heat and Cold for possible moxibustion, the tongue is the first indicator, the pulse is a second indicator, and the patient's desire for a hot or cold drink is a third.

Hernia: Seven direct moxa cones on Liver 1 *Dadun*. Moxa cones for this treatment are about the size of a mung bean.

Chronic cough: Three direct moxa cones on Ren 22 *Tiantu*.

Hiccup: Ren 12 *Zhongwan*. A white tongue coating will indicate Deficiency and the presence of Cold in the Stomach.

Kyphosis (humpback): Du 12 *Shenzhu*. "*Shenzhu*" means "the pillar of the body," and it is an important tonic point for weak patients who cannot stand erect.

Severe chronic diarrhea leading to unconsciousness: Indirect moxa was applied for several hours over the triangular area from Stomach 25 *Tianshu* bilaterally, to Ren 4 *Guanyuan*. Next day, the patient regained consciousness and the diarrhea had stopped. On the third day, the patient was released from the hospital.

Severe headache: The patient was a college professor who read and studied all the time. He experienced occasional and slight relief by applying cold water compresses. Treatment was moxibustion on Du 24 *Shenting*. This point is contraindicated on children under 2 years old because of its proximity to the frontoparietal suture.

Severe headache: The patient's cheeks in the zygomatic area changed to a dark green color. She was dizzy, unable to open her eyes, and too tired to talk. Her whole body felt heavy, and she was nauseous. Direct moxa on Gall Bladder 43 *Xiaxi*.

Breech baby: Three rice-grain-size moxa cones on Urinary Bladder 67 *Zhiyin*. This procedure may be also used any time after the beginning of the third trimester of pregnancy to help regulate the fetus's position.

Moxa on the navel is used to treat:

- chronic diarrhea
- diarrhea and vomiting occurring together
- dysentery
- deep feeling of cold
- abdominal pain
- borborygmus
- urinary incontinence
- urine retention
- rectal prolapse
- swelling, edema
- poor digestion
- infertility
- deficient type stroke

Moxibustion on the navel and the surrounding area is one of the primary methods for promoting the circulation of *qi*.

Since moxibustion is so good for raising the body's resistance, it is fitting to close with a few prescriptions that fortify general health and strengthen immunity.

Du 14 *Dazhui* and **Ren 4** *Guanyuan*. This is an ancient moxa prescription for Reinforcing the Yin and Yang of the whole body. One of this prescription's uses in modern times is to help cancer patients recover from the side effects of chemotherapy.

Gall Bladder 39 *Xuanzhong*. Moxibustion on this point stimulates the production of T cells. *Xuanzhong* also is the Influential Point for marrow, making this point very useful for treating leukemia and chemotherapy patients.

Du 14 *Dazhui*, **Ren 8** *Shenque*, **Stomach 36** *Zusanli*, and **Gall Bladder 39** *Xuanzhong* for treating HIV patients.

And finally, one last prescription for good health from my mentor and dear friend, Dr. Andrew Tseng:

Eat well: do not eat too much spicy food,
or rich, greasy food; do not drink too much alcohol.
Live a peaceful, restful life, and be happy.

Index

— C —

— D —

— E —

— F —

— G-H —

— I-J —

— M —

— N —

— P —

— Q —

— R-S —

— T —

— U-V-W —

About the author:

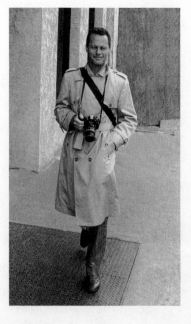

After graduating from the San Francisco College of Acupuncture and Oriental Medicine, Robert Johns earned his doctorate from SAMRA University of Oriental Medicine in Los Angeles, California. Dr. Johns has apprenticed with such masters as Dr. Andrew Tseng, a former District Physician of Shanghai, and Dr. Fung Fung, an herbalist with over sixty years' clinical experience and author of *Sixty Years in Search of Cures*. He has also apprenticed with Dr. Zhu Qi Xiu, Chief of Ophthalmology at the Foshan 2nd Hospital, and has studied with Dr. Ouyang Qun, Vice Chairman of China's National Acupuncture Research Committee.

Since 1984, Dr. Johns has taught traditional Chinese medicine in the San Francisco Bay Area at the San Francisco College of Acupuncture and Oriental Medicine, San Francisco State University, the American College of Traditional Chinese Medicine, The Meiji College of Oriental Medicine, and the University of California at San Francisco. He is licensed as a Qi Gong instructor by Beijing Peoples' University and presently maintains a private practice in Berkeley, California.